The Palliative Care and Hospice Caregiver's Workbook

Sharing the journey with the dying

Lura L. Pethtel M.Ed.
Co-Founder
Institute for Professionalism Inquiry
Summa Health System

and

John D. Engel Ph.D.
Scientific Director
Institute for Professionalism Inquiry
Summa Health System

Foreword by

Timothy Quill M.D.
Professor of Medicine, Psychiatry, and Medical Humanities
Director, Center for Palliative Care and Clinical Ethics
University of Rochester School of Medicine and Dentistry

Radcliffe Publishing
Oxford • New York

Radcliffe Publishing Ltd
18 Marcham Road
Abingdon
Oxon OX14 1AA
United Kingdom

www.radcliffepublishing.com
Electronic catalogue and worldwide online ordering facility.

British Library Cataloguing in Publication Data

A catalogue record for this book is available from the British Library.

ISBN-13: 978 184619 384 2

Typeset by Phoenix Photosetting, Chatham, Kent

Contents

The *Educator's Guide* can be downloaded from
www.radcliffepublishing.com/edguidepalcare

Foreword

Participating in the care of seriously ill, potentially dying patients and their families is not for the fainthearted or for those who are uncurious about themselves or others. On the other hand, there is no better opportunity to learn about the human condition and about the potential for human connection than to voluntarily join with patients and their families in this journey. Of course, patients and families do not have a choice about traveling this path. However, those who make the commitment to travel with them have the opportunity not only to make a difference to those for whom they are caring, but also to grow and evolve themselves as human beings.

Many are drawn to this work because of losses they have experienced in their own lives. Past personal experiences of loss and death can provide a valuable background and important internal resource to identify and empathize with patients and families who are going through this in real time. However, that same experience can also cause lack of objectivity, confusion and distortion between the patient's and family's experience and one's own. It is therefore critical to explore one's own experience in considerable depth before trying to engage in a therapeutic way with critically ill patients and their families.

Considerable self-awareness and self-knowledge are needed to embark on this work. Unfortunately, relatively few clinicians, much less volunteers, have had sufficient training to be fully effective. Good will, dedication, altruism, and enthusiasm are helpful qualities, but they are insufficient in themselves. The kind of learning that is required is a mix of understanding and exploring one's own personal experience of illness, loss and death, as well as understanding how one's views about life and death influence one's behavior and thinking. It also requires learning how to separate one's own experience, values, and biases from those of the patients and families with whom one is working. Finally, trainees must also learn more about how to take care of themselves while they are maintaining engagement with others.

This workbook, which has been prepared by Lura Pethtel and John Engel from the Institute for Professionalism Inquiry of Summa Health System, is the best resource I have seen for guiding teachers and learners in this complex training process. The workbook Units include elements of mindfulness, narrative medicine, appreciative inquiry, and reading provocative articles such that the learners over time come to understand the origins of their own views, values, and biases about death and dying, as well as aspects of what it means to be a caregiver. Participants will also learn about and experiment with modern methods of communication, compassionate presence, and partnering with seriously ill patients and their families. This training gains depth each session, such that learners will emerge from the process more self-aware and more capable of genuine engagement when they eventually join with patients and families in this remarkable process.

Those hospice and palliative care programs that are serious about making sure that their trainees have sufficient self-awareness to be able to compassionately engage with patients and families would do well to consider using these exercises in their training processes. They can be used for training volunteers, hospice nurses, and social workers, as well as physicians. These exercises would also be useful for hospice and palliative care fellows, or for clinicians who are transitioning to this work from other fields. The beauty of the workbook is that each of the Units is a self-contained workshop which can be used in isolation, but the maximum impact of the training would be achieved by completing all of the sessions, since they are well thought out and incremental, each building on preceding sessions and covering an important aspect of the work. These exercises would also be useful for palliative care or hospice teams to go through together as part of their ongoing professional development.

So, many thanks to Lura Pethtel and John Engel for providing us with such a thoughtful guide. I predict that those of you who try it with your staff and trainees will find that it bears fruit not only for your patients and their families, but also for the sustenance and personal development of the staff members themselves.

Timothy Quill, M.D.
Professor of Medicine, Psychiatry, and Medical Humanities
Director, Center for Palliative Care and Clinical Ethics
University of Rochester School of Medicine and Dentistry
March 2010

About the Authors

Lura L. Pethtel M.Ed. During her long tenure at the Northeastern Ohio Universities College of Medicine, Lura served as Associate Dean and taught in the areas of behavioral sciences and humanities, and co-directed courses in spirituality and medicine and in hospice and palliative care. She is a co-founder of the Institute for Professionalism Inquiry, Summa Health System, where she coordinates research and evaluation activities as well as the Humanism and the Healing Arts conference series, and serves as co-director and faculty for the Narrative Medicine course for family medicine residents. Lura worked with the Last Acts organization on a hospice lay volunteer training program, trained more than 100 lay pastoral care volunteers for the Summa Health System, and has conducted workshops on spirituality and health, and spirituality in healthcare and in the workplace. She has served as pastoral care volunteer in the hospital's intensive-care unit, and currently is on call as a *vigil volunteer* in the palliative care unit. She is co-author of several journal articles and, most recently, with colleagues of the Institute for Professionalism Inquiry, she co-authored the book *Narrative in Health Care: Healing Patients, Practitioners, Profession, and Community*.

John D. Engel Ph.D. John, a social scientist, is Scientific Director at the Institute for Professionalism Inquiry, Summa Health System, and Professor Emeritus of Behavioral Science, Northeastern Ohio Universities College of Medicine. His research interests are the philosophy of social science inquiry, qualitative methodology, narrative healthcare, integrating humanities and social sciences with health professions education and practice, and care of the dying. He has taught courses in hospice and palliative care, and has also attended several dying family members and close friends. John has served as founding associate editor for *Qualitative Health Research* and edited the methodology section of that journal. He has been a member of the editorial board of *Evaluation and the Health Professions* since its inception. He has published extensively in his areas of interest, and is currently engaged in conducting a longitudinal study of professional development as well as a participatory action project on the impact of narrative practice in a department of family medicine. His most recent book, *Narrative in Health Care: Healing Patients, Practitioners, Profession, and Community*, was published with colleagues at the Institute for Professionalism Inquiry.

Acknowledgements

We wish to express our gratitude to the countless students, patients, friends, and families who, throughout the years, have shared their lives with us and have been our remarkable and gracious teachers. We give special thanks to Elizabeth Armstrong, and to Drs. Peter Ways, Elizabeth Young, and Timothy Quill, who devoted precious time to reviewing and editing this work, and to Drs. Agnes Csikos, Joseph Zarconi, and Sally Missimi, who partner with us in our endeavors. We are immensely grateful that our friend and colleague, Dr. Robert Blacklow, saw reason to support and promote our early projects which laid the path to this time and work.

To Joe Aulino, our dear friend and soul mate,
who showed us how to both live and die well.

There comes a time
when sea and land
come to rest.
There comes a time
when even the heavens withdraw.
There comes a time
when weary travelers
need a rest from the journey.

Rumi

Part 1:
Getting Started

This program begins by attending to issues that are important for the success of your training, and getting acquainted with your trainer(s) and with your colleagues who also wish to serve the dying. You will learn about the historical shift in how and where people die, the basic functions of modern-day hospice and palliative care, and the roles and functions of professional and lay caregivers. Finally, you will engage in a readers' theater – a play that will enable you to be a companion to Ivan Ilyich on his dying journey.

Unit 1.1: Gaining Perspectives

KEY ISSUES

Modern medicine and technology, hospice, palliative care, palliative care team.

> *To do this work, one must be both a romantic and a realist, both a guide and a student, and most of all, a committed partner.*
>
> Timothy Quill, M.D. (1:31)

INTRODUCTION

The important work that you will be doing depends on your learning and/or strengthening the skills that are critical for a successful caregiver. In our previous experience with training groups such as this, we learned that participants form strong bonds which ultimately serve to foster trust and authenticity as they work through the exercises together. Getting acquainted with your trainer(s) and with your colleagues is the first step in this process. This Unit also provides you with a brief perspective on how end-of-life care has changed over time, and offers you the opportunity, through a readers' theater,* to commonly experience the dying process of one individual.

EXERCISES

A. (35 minutes) *Taking Care of Business*

The trainer will introduce him- or herself and provide you with instructions about such matters as room assignments, schedule, seating arrangements, parking availability, and so forth. Then, in turn, each participant should state their name and where they live. **Do not provide any other information at this time**.

* A readers' theater is a play in which lines are not memorized by actors, but instead are read by group participants.

B. (30 minutes) *Introduction to the Training Program*

One or more volunteers should read aloud *About this Educational Guide* provided below. Take this opportunity to ask questions about the program and express any concerns that you may have.

About This Educational Guide

This educational guide has been designed as a training program for small groups of individuals who wish to volunteer in hospice or palliative care settings and who have the benefit of a trainer. Professional caregivers who want to strengthen their skills, and relatives or friends who anticipate attending to a dying person will also find it valuable, even though they may not fully engage in some of the exercises that require group participation. It does not encompass the physical/medical aspects of the dying process, but rather it focuses on the skills and abilities that are critical in establishing a compassionate relationship with a dying person and assisting them with psycho-social-spiritual issues.

The guide has been formatted as a paper–pencil workbook organized into five Parts that provide a comprehensive and sequential learning program. It comprises 16 separate but related Units, each constructed to be approximately 180 minutes long. Every Unit begins with a listing of key issues, a quieting exercise, and the sharing of a reflective journal note based on the activities in the previous Unit. (Please note that this first Unit does not include either a "quieting exercise" or a "journal note.") This material is followed by introductory material and skill exercises. Each Unit ends with an assignment for the next session (some have been written into the Guide and some will be determined by the trainer), additional resources (when relevant), and a reference section.

A variety of learning experiences have been employed, including large and small group activities, discussion, close reading, creative writing, self-exploration, and skill development and practice. Selected prose and poems that are relevant to the context have been included throughout. The skills that we introduce are fundamental and extremely important for the successful caregiver.

Organization

Part 1: Getting Started provides participants with the opportunity to learn about the program and become acquainted with their trainer(s) and colleagues. A brief essay describes the historical shift in how and where people die, and covers basic functions of modern-day hospice, palliative care, and caregiving teams. Participants will engage in a readers' theater. Part 1 contains just one Unit:

- Gaining Perspectives.

Part 2: Understanding the Caregiver's Self provides exercises and activities that enable participants to explore and come to terms with their own feelings about dying and death. This Part contains six Units:

- Reflecting on Death
- Mindfulness
- Self-Knowledge
- Spiritual Knowledge
- The Whole Self: Body–Mind–Spirit
- Facing Death.

Part 3: Understanding Ourselves in Service of the Dying Person focuses on the many influences in our lives and how they shape our personhood and beliefs and how we deal with life losses. This Part contains three Units:

- Social and Cultural Influences
- Spiritual and Religious Influences
- The Nature of Loss and Suffering.

Part 4: Ways of Helping the Dying Person focuses on effective communication and the essential skills of mindful listening and responding with empathy and compassion. This Part contains five Units:

- Fundamentals of Communication
- Compassionate Presence, Mindful Listening, and Effective Responding
- Fears and Assumptions About Death
- Narratives of Suffering
- Expressive Activities that Aid in Relieving Suffering.

Part 5: Honoring the Caregiver emphasizes the need for self-care and provides an opportunity for trainees to conduct a self-check for readiness to begin the journey with a dying person. This Part contains just one Unit:

- Nurture and Honor Yourself!

Guidelines for Participants

The skills that we introduce in this guide are fundamental and essential for the role of caregiver. However, just like learning to ride a bike or play a musical instrument, the skills must be practiced correctly, regularly, and consistently. Not only are they important for caregiving, but they are also life skills that will help participants to build and improve both their personal and professional relationships. You may find that you already possess many of the skills which are important for this work. If this is true for you, make this a time to review and refresh your skills and help your colleagues to develop theirs. Others of you may feel that you still have a long way to go, so you should take full advantage of this opportunity to learn. Individual caregivers and friends or relatives who use this guide should read each Part and Unit carefully and attempt to complete each exercise.

In order to be fully prepared as knowledgeable and effective caregivers, trainees are strongly advised to attend all sessions, to participate fully and openly, and to demonstrate compassion, genuineness, honesty, and acceptance of the opinions, beliefs, and values of others. Participants should be willing to ask questions, absorb new information and consciously practice techniques. **Learning will be greatly enhanced through the willingness of all participants to self-explore and share their thoughts and feelings, and to help others to do the same.**

Throughout the program, participants will be asked to read aloud and discuss each element of the Unit, including the opening quote, the introduction, and any poems or prose that are located in the Unit. **Beginning with the very first session, we cannot over-emphasize the need for participants to maintain confidentiality throughout this work with colleagues and later while attending a dying person. The sharing of intimate information is highly unethical.**

Program Learning Objectives

1. Develop and/or strengthen the knowledge, skills, attitudes, and behaviors that are essential for effective caregiving.
2. Understand and commit to the importance of confidentiality.
3. Develop mindfulness.
4. Examine our own current attitude, assumptions, and concerns about death.
5. Learn to explore the needs of the dying person with respect and compassion.
6. Develop and strengthen self-awareness and identify personal needs and goals for personal growth.
7. Examine the many influences in our lives.
8. Develop effective communication skills.
9. Examine our own spiritual beliefs and how they affect our life.
10. Discern the body–mind–spirit interconnections.
11. Become knowledgeable about the differing spiritual beliefs and practices among human beings.
12. Develop an understanding of the effects of loss and the nature of suffering and grief.
13. Explore the ways of dying and the many changes and needs that may arise during the dying process.

14. Learn and practice techniques that may alleviate suffering.
15. Explore ways to care for ourselves while caring for another.

C. (40 minutes) *Getting Acquainted*

Take about 5 minutes to complete the Biosketch below. Please write legibly so that someone else will be able to read it. Form pairs. Give your Biosketch to your partner. Take 2 to 3 minutes to study their sketch and then discuss it briefly. You may wish to clarify some points with this individual. Then, using the sketch and any notes that you have, introduce your partner to the group.

Name ______________________________

Home town/city ______________________________

Family make-up ______________________________

Ethnic background ______________________________

Religious affiliation (if any) ______________________________

Educational background ______________________________

____

Work, place(s) of employment ______________________________

____

Interests, hobbies, activities, etc. ______________________________

____

Reasons for taking this training ______________________________

____

____

Strengths you bring to this training ______________________________

D. (30 minutes) *The Dying Process in Modern Times*

The trainer will ask for volunteers to share the reading of this short essay. Discuss key issues in the large group and ask any questions you may have.

> *The word death is not pronounced in New York, in Paris, in London, because it burns the lips. The Mexican, in contrast, is familiar with death, jokes about it, caresses it, sleeps with it, celebrates it; it is one of his favorite toys and his most steadfast loves.*
>
> Octavio Paz (1:3)

Throughout time and all cultures, the suffering and dying have sought the help of healers. Healing, as discussed by Michael Kearney (2: ixx), is a "process of becoming psychologically and spiritually more integrated and whole; a phenomenon which enables persons to become more completely themselves and more fully alive." Prior to the twentieth century, people in the Western world believed that caring for the dying occurred in the home. The sick and dying were taken care of primarily by family members and friends, or sometimes by hired caregivers. During the early twentieth century, with the rise of hospitals, dying became a medical event and most people in Europe and North America went to hospital to die. By the mid-1970s, more than 70% of deaths occurred in hospital settings. The shift in location of dying had an impact on the nature of dying. Too often, people's experiences in these institutions were dehumanizing. In these settings, family members were "guests" and control of care rested with unknown healthcare professionals. It must also be noted that, during this period, dying was a relatively brief affair; few experienced prolonged states of severe incapacity and dependence.

As modern medicine became more scientific and as the use of medical technology increased during the mid twentieth century, the goal of medicine shifted towards the identification and cure of disease. The purpose of medicine became the prolongation of life through the use of increased technological intervention and advanced pharmacopeias. Most notable among these technological interventions were the techniques of resuscitation and advanced life support that led to the development and widespread proliferation of cardiopulmonary resuscitation (CPR) and intensive-care units (ICUs) during the 1960s (3). In addition, with the development of sophisticated drug therapies, infectious diseases were often "conquered." News of these advances was generally heralded by the media, with a public fanfare. To be sure, this was appropriate in many instances. However, an unexpected outcome of these events was the evolution of a "cult of cure" among the public (4).

One impact of the development of modern medicine and medical technology concerns the way in which people get sick and die today compared with what occurred during previous periods of medicine. Hallenback (3: 2) notes:

> In 1900 the top five causes of death in the United States were respiratory infections (influenza and pneumonia), tuberculosis, gastroenteritis, heart disease, and stroke, in that order. With the exception of tuberculosis, most deaths were relatively sudden, occurring over a few days of illness. In 2000 the top five causes of death in the United States were heart disease, cancer, stroke, chronic obstructive pulmonary disease (COPD) and accidents. With the exception of sudden heart attacks and accidental deaths, most of these deaths were due to prolonged, chronic illness.

In many instances, modern ways of becoming sick and dying have not only overwhelmed institutions' ability to care in humane ways for the dying, but also hidden the fact that it is often difficult to die. Iona Heath (5:41) notes:

> The transition from a strong healthy body to one capable of slipping gently into death is hard. Unless it is the result of sudden and overwhelming catastrophe, the transition cannot be achieved without experiencing fatigue and weakness and other physical symptoms of debility and decline.

As a response to our modern forms of sickness and ways of dying, two important developments have occurred, namely hospice and palliative care.

The roots of hospice began in the sixth century. Buddhists established a network of medical centers across India. Monks at these temples often diagnosed and cared for the sick and dying. For over 2500 years, Buddhists have contemplated how to live with and make friends with death. In the Western world, the word *hospice* came into being during medieval times. It is derived from the Latin word *hospes* meaning "guest" or "host." Travel-weary and battle-worn crusaders returning from the Holy Land found respite in monasteries which, among other things, became places for the sick and dying.

The modern hospice movement is generally associated with the work of two women, Dame Cicely Saunders and Elisabeth Kubler-Ross. Dame Saunders, a British physician and former nurse and social worker, founded St. Christopher's Hospice in London in 1967 after working tirelessly with the dying for many years. Based on her experiences with the dying she knew that it was critical to focus on better pain management in end-of-life care, and to recognize that the dying are whole people with social, psychological, emotional, and spiritual needs (6). In the spring of 1965, Saunders was a visiting faculty member at Yale University's School of Nursing. This contact was influential in sowing the seeds of the hospice philosophy and practice in the U.S.A.

The other notable person in the hospice movement, Elisabeth Kubler-Ross, had conducted a series of conversations with dying patients at a Chicago hospital (7). Through her studies, she developed an elaborate description of a series of stages that she believed were a part of the dying person's experience, namely denial, anger, bargaining, depression, and acceptance.* Her work contributed a great deal to our knowledge of dying. In 1972, she testified at the first national hearings on dying and death conducted by the U.S. Senate Special Committee on Aging. Kubler-Ross promoted the need for dignity during the dying process, and her efforts were instrumental in stimulating the growth of hospice in North America.

Despite early resistance, the medical establishment came to accept hospice and the benefits that its volunteers provide to patients and their families. Derek Doyle, medical director at St. Columba's Hospice in Edinburgh, Scotland, notes (8:8):

> The word 'hospice' is now a hallowed one, accepted into our language, but to doctors and nurses a more accurate description (and the one usually used by them) is a palliative care unit. This better defines their role – the care of people with "active, progressive, far-advanced illness who have a relatively short life left to them and their need to be guaranteed the best possible quality of remaining life", something achieved by highly skilled attention to every aspect of their physical, emotional, social, and spiritual suffering by a closely integrated team of professionals. They are there to relieve suffering, not to prolong life. They recognize they cannot cure but they can, in a thousand ways, continue to care. They set out neither to extend nor abbreviate life.

The first hospices in North America provided an alternative to traditional hospitals in care of the dying. By 1975, hospices were established in Connecticut, New York, and Montreal (3, 8, 9). All were inpatient units and were funded with a combination of grants and donations. Today hospice is both a philosophy of care and a set of integrated services. Although many private for-profit agencies do exist, most services are supported by the U.S. government through Medicare and are found in both patients' homes and inpatient units

* These stages are currently thought to be good signposts to sensitize caregivers to what a dying person might experience, rather than a set of immutable periods that each person must go through in the specified order.

in various healthcare institutions (e.g. hospitals, nursing facilities, assisted or independent living settings). A significant amount of home hospice care is provided to the dying person by a family member or other loved one serving as the hands-on caregiver.

As a philosophy of care, hospice recognizes death as a normal and final stage of life. Hospice implements this view by supporting patients to continue an alert, pain-free life (as much as possible) by managing symptoms so that their last days may be spent with emotional support, dignity, and quality as they are surrounded by family and other loved ones. Hospice care is provided by a team-oriented group of specially prepared professionals (including physicians, nurses, social workers, and clergy), volunteers, and family members.

Whereas hospice in the U.S. focuses on relieving symptoms and supporting patients with a life expectancy of usually about six months or less, palliative care may be provided at any time during a serious or life-threatening illness. The term "palliation" derives from the Latin word *palliare*, which means to "cloak" or "shield." Palliative care shields the patient from the symptoms of serious illness whether or not the illness is terminal, and may be provided alongside curative care. Thus hospice programs always provide palliative care for patients who are no longer seeking curative care, but, in general, not all palliative care programs focus on the terminally ill. However, it is important to note that such distinctions between hospice and palliative care are becoming blurred as the need for the appropriate interface between these two approaches is recognized. In general, in the face of serious illness, as the benefits of curative care diminish, the benefits of palliative care increase, and at the point of a prognosis of limited life expectancy, hospice services, including palliative care, become critical for the patient. The palliative care team (physicians, nurses, social workers, clergy, and volunteers) provides treatment of pain and other symptoms, management of the disease and any treatment complications, help in navigating complex healthcare systems, guidance with difficult and complex treatment alternatives, practical information and assistance, and emotional and spiritual support of the dying (10–12).

ADDITIONAL RESOURCES

1. Byock I. *Dying Well: peace and possibilities at the end of life*. New York: Riverhead Books; 1997.
2. Quill TE. *Caring for Patients at the End of Life: facing an uncertain future together.* New York: Oxford University Press; 2001.
3. Snyder C, Quill TE, eds. *Physician's Guide to End-of-Life Care*. Philadelphia, PA: American College of Physicians; 2001.
4. www.DyingWell.org

REFERENCES

1. Octavio Paz, Mexican poet and critic. In: SL Bertman (ed.) *Facing Death: images, insights, and interventions*. Bristol, PA: Taylor and Francis; 1991.
2. Kearney M. *A Place of Healing: working with suffering in living and dying*. New York: Oxford University Press; 2000.
3. Hallenback JL. *Palliative Care Perspectives*. New York: Oxford University Press; 2003.
4. Goulb E. *The Limits of Medicine: how science shapes our hope for the cure*. New York: Times Books; 1994.
5. Heath I. *Matters of Life and Death: key writings*. Oxford: Radcliffe Publishing; 2008.
6. Du Boulay S. *Cicely Saunders*. London: Hodder & Stoughton; 1994.
7. Kubler-Ross E. *On Death and Dying*. New York: Macmillan; 1969.
8. Doyle D. *Caring for a Dying Relative: a guide for families*. New York: Oxford University Press; 1994.
9. Stoddard S. *The Hospice Movement*. New York: Vintage; 1992.
10. Abel EK. The hospice movement: institutionalizing innovation. *Int J Health Serv*. 1986; **16:** 71–85.
11. www.Getpalliativecare.org (2009, Center to Advance Palliative Care).
12. Foley KM, Gelband H, eds. *Improving Palliative Care for Cancer: summary and recommendations*. Washington, D.C.: National Academy Press; 2001.

E. (50 minutes) *The Death of Ivan Ilyich: A Readers' Theater*

We have chosen to adapt Leo Tolstoy's widely read classic novella, *The Death of Ivan Ilyich*, as a readers' theater. The purpose of conducting a readers' theater is to invite you to serve as readers in performing this play and then to discuss the issues that are raised. A volunteer should first read the paragraph about Tolstoy at the top of the title page. Each participant should volunteer to read one (or more) of the 10 spoken parts. The narrator's part requires a strong reader.

Tolstoy was born in 1828 into a long line of Russian nobility. He married at the age of 34, but the marriage was soon plagued with tension and unhappiness. Later in his life he suffered serious self-doubt and depression, and even became suicidal. This prompted a period of intense spiritual introspection which resulted in his conversion to a Christian/Buddhist belief system. Prior to his death he struggled with his identity. He regretted his actions from decades earlier and how he had lived and who he had become. Tolstoy died in 1910.

THE DEATH OF IVAN ILYCH*

By

Count Leo Tolstoy

Adapted for Readers' Theater by Lura Pethtel and John D. Engel

CAST

****

Narrator
Ivan Ilyich Golovin
Praskovia Feodorovna Golovin (Ivan's wife)
Liza (Ivan's daughter)
Vassili (Ivan's son, no spoken part)
Gerasim (house servant)
Lacofsky (Ivan's brother-in-law)
Piotr Ivanovitch (colleague)
Feodor Vasilyevitch (colleague)
Leschititsky (eminent doctor)
Nikolaef (ordinary doctor)
Piotr (the footman, no spoken part)

Scene 1

Narrator: The time and setting for our story is nineteenth-century Russia. We begin by hearing about Ivan Ilyich Golovin's career in the years preceding his death.

For many years since his graduation from law school, Ivan had enjoyed a highly successful professional life as a magistrate of the courts, with continual promotions and assignments in various locations. At the time of his death he was serving a ministry in Petersburg.

Early in his career Ivan had married Praskovia Feodorovna Mikhel, who came from good aristocratic stock and was sweet, intelligent, pretty, and eminently respectable. The beginning of their married life was blissful until Praskovia first became pregnant, and with the birth of additional children she grew increasingly jealous, demanding of Ivan's attention,

* Adapted from *The Death of Ivan Ilyich*, translated from the Russian version by Nathan Haskell Dole. Copyright 1887 by Thomas Y. Crowell & Company, New York.

and disagreeable and generally disruptive of their pleasant lifestyle. The death of two of their children severely compounded the situation. The more irritating and demanding his wife became, the more Ivan transferred the center of gravity of his life to his work, and the more ambitious he became. Soon his life focused on his work, the consciousness of his own power and the importance of his success in the eyes of high and low. Unfortunately, yet another child died, leaving only his daughter, Liza, now 16, and his young schoolboy son, Vasilli. So it was that Ivan lived for several more years.

At the news of his death, Ivan's colleagues, who knew he had been ill for several weeks with an incurable disease, began thinking of their own probable career advancements now that a vacancy had opened. The closest of his friends were Vasilyevitch and Ivanovitch.

Feodor Vasilyevitch: Now I'll probably get Shtabel's place or Vinnikof's. It's been promised to me for a long time. What was the matter with Ivan Ilyich?

Piotr Ivanovitch: Each of his doctors thought something different. The last time I saw him, I thought he was getting better. Yes, now that he is gone, I'll have to put in for my brother-in-law's transfer from Kaluga. My wife will be very pleased, and no one can say I never did anything for her relatives. But since I have been friends with Ivan since law school, I feel an obligation to him. I will attend his funeral.

Narrator: Piotr Ivanovitch entered the Ilyich residence with a feeling of uncertainty as to how to behave under such circumstances. He began to cross himself as he moved toward the coffin. As he did, he noticed the servant Gerasim, who Ivan was very fond of, sprinkling something on the floor to mask the faint odor of decomposition. Just before the funeral was to begin, Praskovia took Ivanovitch aside.

Praskovia: I have some business with you. Ivan Ilyich suffered dreadfully in his last days. Oh, it was terrible! For three days and nights he screamed without stopping. It was unbearable. I can't understand how I survived it. How I suffered!

Narrator: Ivanovitch thought to himself.

Ivanovitch: Three days and nights of appalling suffering and death. Why that could happen to me, too, at any time. But thinking such thoughts is not good for me, I must think of other things.

Narrator: Weeping, Praskovia continued to speak to Ivanovitch of her primary concern, which was how she could extract more money out of the Treasury on her husband's death. After considering the situation, Ivanovitch said that he believed that nothing more could be done.

When Ivanovitch entered the funeral room he met Ivan's beautiful young daughter,

Liza. She was dressed in black and wore a gloomy, almost irritated expression. Behind her stood her fiancé, also a magistrate, a wealthy young man with a similar offended expression. Ivanovitch then caught sight of Ivan's small schoolboy son, who looked very much like Ivan. He saw that Vassili's eyes were tearstained.

Scene 2

Narrator: The early years of married life were difficult. Praskovia had become quarrelsome and irritating. As this happened, Ivan withdrew more and more into his work. But there were many stressful times at work and after losing one position, due to a political conflict, he was fortunate to gain an excellent position in Petersburg. Relations with his wife improved somewhat, in part because of this new position and the social advantage it brought with it. When Ivan and his family had first arrived in Petersburg, they had secured an excellent apartment, exactly what he and his wife dreamed of. He personally oversaw the decorations, and at times did some of the decorating himself. On just such an occasion, he fell off a ladder and hit his side against the handle of a window. It hurt for a little while but then passed. The new apartment had a distinctly aristocratic flavor, and they had all settled into a harmonious life and courted members of the proper social class at their new home. Ivan Ilyich's pleasures were those of self-love, social vanity, and playing *vint*, a very popular card game of the social elite.

When Ivan Ilyich's illness first began, he complained of a strange taste in his mouth and something that felt not quite right on the left side of his stomach. Then the discomfort began to increase – not yet quite pain, but an awareness of a permanent heaviness in his side. He fell into a poor state of mind which grew stronger and began to spoil the light, much more pleasant way of life just established in the Golovin household. Now it was he, Ivan, who most often started the quarreling, and generally at the moment he started eating. He began to blame Praskovia for everything.

Praskovia: Ivan Ilyich, it is fortunate that I was blessed with such a sweet nature to put up with your difficult character and horrible temper all these years. As for your illness, I believe you must have a constitutional disorder prompted by food.

Narrator: Praskovia decided her husband's appalling character made her life a misery, and the more she pitied herself, the more she loathed her husband. She started wishing he would die, but realized that if he did die there would be no salary, and that made her even more irritated with him.

Praskovia: If you are ill then you should get treatment! I insist that you go to see the eminent physician, Dr. Leschititsky.

Narrator: He went, and everything was as he expected it to be. The waiting, the charade played out by the doctor – the tapping, the listening, the questions requiring futile replies, and the meaningful look which proclaimed, "Come, come, sir, just rely on me and we'll sort it all out." All this was familiar to Ivan. Just as Ivan put on a show in court for the man on trial, so the doctor put on a show for him.

Ivan Ilyich: Only one thing is important to me, Doctor. Is my condition dangerous or not?

Doctor Leschititsky: (*arrogantly*) It is most probable that you are experiencing one of several maladies: a floating kidney, perhaps chronic catarrh, or a disease of the blind gut.

Narrator: For the doctor and quite probably for everyone, his illness didn't matter in the least, but for Ivan it was bad. He began to feel intense pity for himself and great bitterness against the doctor who was so indifferent to a question of such importance.

Ivan Ilyich: (*with disdain*) I imagine we sick people often ask you irrelevant questions. By and large, is it a dangerous illness or not?

Doctor Leschititsky: (*arrogantly*) I have already told you what I deem necessary and appropriate. Further evidence will come from the analyses (the doctor bows him out).

Narrator: On the way home, Ivan tried to make sense of all the scientific language used by the doctor. He found everything and everyone along the way to be gloomy. At home, in the middle of his account of his doctor's visit to his wife, his daughter, Liza, came in with her hat on as she was about to go out with her mother. With effort she sat down to listen to this tedious stuff. She could not contain herself for long, and her mother also stopped listening.

Praskovia: (*offhandedly*) Well, I'm delighted! I'll send Gerasim to the pharmacy. Now mind you, take the medicine properly.

Ivan Ilyich: Well, who knows, perhaps it really is nothing much.

Narrator: Ivan became totally preoccupied with his illness and following the prescribed treatment. The pain grew no less, but he made great efforts to persuade himself that he felt better, and for a time he was able to deceive himself until something went wrong. Then he immediately felt the full force of the disease. He despaired.

Ivan Ilyich: (*raging*) I was just getting better. The medicine was finally beginning to work. These people are killing me. I need peace of mind. All this disruption infuriates me. The more I read the medical books and see the doctors, the worse I feel.

Narrator: He went to several more specialists, but their diagnoses and advice only served to confuse Ivan further and confirm his doubts. He lost faith in all the physicians and fell into profound gloom. Then a lady of his acquaintance suggested something new – that his sickness could surely be cured by the powerful icons that are known to heal. He found himself believing this, and that horrified him.

Ivan Ilyich: I mustn't give in to hypochondria. I must choose one doctor and keep strictly to his course of treatment. That's what I'll do! Enough of this dithering.

Narrator: It was easy to say and impossible to do. The pain in his side seemed to grow steadily worse and was wearing him down. The taste in his mouth grew more peculiar, and his strength and appetite were both diminishing. He could no longer deceive himself. Something very significant was taking place inside him. And he was the only one who knew about it. None around him understood or cared. They thought that everything was going on as usual. This was what tormented Ivan more than anything.

His wife and daughter, who were caught up in their social whirl, were irritated by how demanding and cheerless he was, as though this were their fault.

Praskovia would say to her friends, "You know, one day Ivan takes the drops and eats what he's ordered and goes to bed in good time. The next day, if I don't keep an eye on him, he forgets to take anything, he eats anything and stays up way too late for his card game."

Ivan Ilyich: What difference does staying up to play cards make? I can't sleep because of the pain.

Praskovia: What nonsense! You'll never get well like this. You'll just go on making us miserable. You are to blame for your illness, and this whole business is greatly unpleasant for me.

Narrator: Ivan believed his coworkers had also developed a curious attitude toward him, like he was soon to vacate his post. Even at his card games he became befuddled and his friends grew silent and gloomy. Ivan felt now as though poison permeated his whole existence, and that he poisoned the lives of others. With this knowledge and with his physical pain and his terror, Ivan spent most nights sleepless, and then in the morning rose only to go through it all again. Every minute of every day was torment.

Ivan Ilyich: Why must I live in this way, on the very edge of destruction, without a single being who might understand and pity me?

Scene 3

Narrator: In mid-winter, Lacofsky came to visit. Upon seeing Ivan for the first time, he opened his mouth to gasp and just stopped himself. That movement confirmed it all for Ivan.

Ivan Ilyich: What? Have I changed?

Lacofsky: Yes, there is a change.

Narrator: Later, Ivan saw that the door to Praskovia's sitting room was shut. He tiptoed up to it and listened.

Praskovia: Nonsense, you're exaggerating.

Lacofsky: What do you mean, exaggerating? You can't see it? He's a dead man, look at his eyes. There's no light in them. What's wrong with him, anyway?

Praskovia: No one knows. Nikolaef, one of the doctors, said something, but I don't remember. Leschititsky, the eminent doctor, said the opposite.

Narrator: Ivan Ilyich went into his study, lay down and began thinking. He remembered everything the doctors had told him, how the kidney had torn loose and was floating about. In his imagination he tried to catch his kidney and pin it down and stop it wandering. He decided to go to see Ivanovitch's friend, Doctor Nikolaef, once again.

Doctor Nikolaef: There is some little thing, a minute little something, in the blind gut. It can all get better. It is just a matter of increasing the energy of one organ and diminishing the activity of another. Absorption will take place and everything will get better.

Narrator: Ivan went home and occupied his mind with work. Then guests arrived and Ivan spent the evening in a cheerful manner. Later, he took his leave and went into the small room off his study where he had been sleeping since his illness had begun. He began thinking.

Ivan Ilyich: I can see how the correction of my blind gut can occur. Absorption is taking place, evacuation occurs, correct functioning is re-established. Yes, that's how it should be. We just have to give nature a hand. I just have to take my medicine steadily and avoid adverse influences. Already I feel a little better, a lot better. When I pinch my side it doesn't even hurt. It is really a lot better already. That blind gut is setting itself right, it is becoming absorbed.

Narrator: Suddenly he felt the familiar old, dull, gnawing pain and the familiar disgusting stuff in his mouth. His heart contracted, his head clouded.

Ivan Ilyich: My God! My God! It will never end! It's not a matter of blind gut or the kidney but of life and … death. Yes, there was life and now it's going, it's going, and I can't hold it back. Why should I deceive myself? It is obvious to everyone except me that I'm dying and it's only a question of how many weeks, days, even now, maybe.

I'll be no more and then what will there be? Nothing. Then where will I be, when I will be no longer? Is this really death? Go away, I don't want you. Yes, death. And none of them know and none of them want to know and none of them are sorry. They're having fun. They don't care, but they'll die just like me. Idiocy! Sooner for me, later for them, but it will come. And they're happy. Mindless brutes!

I must calm down and think everything through from the beginning. There was the beginning of the illness. I knocked my side, but was the same before and after. It ached a bit and then a bit more and then there were doctors and then depression, dreariness, doctors again and I kept coming closer and closer to the abyss. And here I am wasted away, no light in my eyes. This is death and I'm thinking about my gut. I'm thinking about putting my kidney right and this is death. Can this really be death?

Narrator: Panic overcame Ivan and he lost his breath. Losing his temper, he knocked over the bedside table. Then, in despair, he fell back expecting instant death. The guests were leaving when Praskovia heard something fall. She went to Ivan's room.

Praskovia: What's the matter?

Ivan Ilyich: Nothing. I knocked the table over by mistake.

Praskovia: You know, I think we should get Leschititsky to visit you here.

Ivan Ilyich: No!

Narrator: Praskovia sat with Ivan a bit longer, then kissed him on the forehead. At that moment, he hated her with all the strength of his soul and had to make an effort not to push her away.

Praskovia: The last guests are leaving. I must go. Goodnight. God give you rest.

Scene 4

Narrator: Deep down Ivan knew he was dying, but he could not understand and he could not accept it.

Ivan Ilyich: It cannot be right for me to die. That would be too terrible. If I had to die, I would have known it; my inner voice would have told me so. Now look! It can't be, but it is. How can it be? How can I understand it? I will find ways to take my mind from all this. I'll get back to work. After all, that was my life. I will forget this thinking about death.

Narrator: He went back to court, chatted with his friends and took his place on the bench as he always had done and opened the proceedings. But suddenly the pain in his side started its business, sucking away at him. *It* came up and stood right in front of him and looked at him and he froze. The light died out of his eyes.

Ivan Ilyich: Surely, *it* can't be the only truth? My court duties can no longer free me from *it*. *It* draws attention to itself. Regardless of what I do to forget, there *it* is, the same thing still crouching there, gnawing away. I can no longer forget, *it* is distinctly staring at me. What is the point of it all?

Narrator: Ivan went home and back to his study to lie down. He was alone with *it* again. Face to face with *it* and nothing to do but look at *it* and grow cold.

Scene 5

Narrator: Imperceptibly, during the third month of Ivan Ilyich's illness, it happened that his wife, his daughter, the servants, his friends, and his doctors and most of all himself understood that their only interest was in how quickly he would die and free the living from the burden of his presence and himself from the suffering. Despite the use of opium and the increased injections of morphine, Ivan slept less and less and the pain increased more and more. But the need to take care of his excretions was the most unbearable. This situation tormented Ivan – the dirt, the indecency, the smell, and the knowledge that another person had to participate. But in his torment, his consolation came to light. It was Gerasim, the peasant who served at the table, who always came to carry out the soil. He was always bright and cheerful. At first Ivan was discomforted by him, but one day after Ivan was getting up from the commode, he was unable to pull up his trousers and fell exhausted into a nearby armchair.

Ivan Ilyich: Gerasim.

Gerasim: Can I do anything for you?

Ivan Ilyich: Please help me. I think it must be unpleasant for you. You must forgive me. I can't help it.

Gerasim: Not at all sir. Why shouldn't I take a little trouble? You're not so well.

Narrator: Gerasim cheerfully removed the pan from the commode and left the room to dispose of it. When he returned a few moments later, Ivan was still in the armchair.

Ivan Ilyich: Gerasim, could you please help me again? Just come over here. Lift me up. It's hard for me on my own.

Gerasim: Of course. Let me just steady you as you stand and then I can adjust your clothing.

Ivan Ilyich: Please take me over to the divan. How lightly and how well you do everything! Move that chair for me, please, under my legs. It's easier for me when my feet are raised. I feel better when my legs are high. Now put that cushion under them.

Narrator: Gerasim did these tasks carefully and with great kindness. It seemed to Ivan that when Gerasim was holding his legs high they felt best, and when placed lower on the cushion the pain returned.

Ivan Ilyich: Gerasim, are you busy at the moment?

Gerasim: Not in the least.

Ivan Ilyich: What have you still got to do?

Gerasim: What me? I've nothing to do, I've done it all – there's only the wood to chop for tomorrow.

Ivan Ilyich: Then hold my legs up high, could you?

Gerasim: Of course I can.

Ivan Ilyich: But what about the firewood?

Gerasim: Don't worry about that, sir. We'll find time.

Narrator: Ivan Ilyich asked Gerasim to sit down and hold his legs, and talk to him. It all seemed to make him feel better while Gerasim was holding up his legs. From that time on, Ivan Ilyich began calling for him occasionally. Gerasim held his legs up willingly and talked to him with a lightness, with a simplicity and kindness that touched Ivan Ilyich. He was offended by healthy and good spirits in everyone else, but Gerasim's strength and cheerfulness soothed him rather than hurt him.

Ivan Ilyich suffered most of all from the lies – the lie that everyone accepted that he was just ill and not dying, that he need only keep calm and take his medicine and something good would happen. But he knew better. There would be only pain and agonizing death. And, most of all, he resented that they forced him to participate in these lies. Somehow, he could not find the courage to say to them "Stop lying!"

Ivan Ilyich: Everyone around me reduces my death to a casual unpleasantness, an offense against propriety. The propriety that I have served all my life. No one pities me because they don't understand my situation. Only Gerasim understands and is sorry for me. Gerasim knows that it is good for me when he holds my legs. And many times he holds my legs on his shoulders for an entire night and doesn't go to bed.

Gerasim: You mustn't worry, your Honor, I'll get sleep another time. With thee so poorly, how couldn't I spare a little trouble? We'll all go someday, why not take a little trouble?

Narrator: After moments of great pain, Ivan wanted someone to pity him like a sick child would be pitied. And while he was ashamed at the thought, he longed to be stroked, kissed, cried over a little. In his relationship with Gerasim there was something like this, and consequently this relationship brought Ivan great comfort.

Scene 6

Narrator: Piotr, the footman, came in to blow out the candles. It was the only way that Ivan Ilyich knew day from night. In the haze of pain, all blended together – day and night, days of the week, the comings and goings of people. Piotr offered Ivan some tea, but he declined and asked Piotr to leave. However, as Piotr started to leave, Ivan became fearful of being alone and asked him to return, thinking that he might try some tea and some medicine.

Ivan Ilyich: Piotr, give me my medicine. You never know, maybe the medicine might still help. My mouth tastes terrible. No, it won't help, that's all rubbish and lies. Look here, the dreadful, sickly, hopeless taste in my mouth has returned. No, I can't believe it anymore. That pain, that pain, I wish it would ease even just for a minute. Oh, Piotr, just bring me the tea.

Narrator: Ivan Ilyich washed his face, brushed his teeth and combed his hair. This last act frightened him. The look of his thin hair clinging to his pallid forehead was gruesome. He dared not look at the rest of his body. Beyond the pain, it was the misery of his existence that caused the most suffering for Ivan.

Just then the door bell rings and it is the doctor. Ivan, sensing who is at the door, makes up his mind that he'll tell the doctor that he can't go on like this and that he must think of something.

Doctor Leschititsky: There you are, all in a panic for some reason, but in a minute we'll make everything right.

Narrator: The doctor breezes in, fresh, brisk, fat, and cheerful. He knows his expression is inappropriate here, but he has put it on once and for all and cannot take it off again, like a man who has put on tails in the morning and driven off to pay a round of calls with no opportunity to change. As he approaches Ivan, he rubs his hands together briskly.

Doctor Leschititsky: My hands are chilly. It's quite a frost. Let me just get warm. Well now, how did you pass the night?

Narrator: Ivan Ilyich looks at the doctor with an expression that asks "Will you never feel ashamed of your lies?" But the doctor does not want to understand his question.

Ivan Ilyich: It's all so dreadful. The pain won't stop, not even for a little. If only there was something.

Doctor Leschititsky: Yes, you sick men always say that. Well now, I think I've got a little warmer. How do you do today?

Narrator: As the doctor sets a serious expression, he starts examining his patient, tapping and listening. Ivan Ilyich knows definitely and indubitably that this is all nonsense, a hollow sham. But he allows himself to be taken in, as in the old days when he gave in to the lawyers' speeches when he knew perfectly well that they were all lying and why they were lying.

Praskovia enters the room, moves to Ivan, and kisses him. Ivan Ilyich scrutinizes her all over, and takes exception to her plump, white, clean hands and neck, her shiny hair and bright eyes, full of life. He detests her with all the strength of his soul. And her touch makes him suffer from his surge of hatred. Her attitude toward him and his illness is still the same. Just as the doctor has worked out an attitude toward his patients which he can no longer shake off, so she has worked out her attitude toward him – that he isn't doing something he ought to be doing, and it's all his fault, while she lovingly reproaches him.

Praskovia: He just won't do as he's told! He will not take the drops on time. But the main thing is, he lies down in a position that must surely be bad for him, with his legs in the air.

Doctor Leschititsky: What are we to do? These invalids sometimes think up the funniest things, but we can forgive them.

Narrator: With the exam completed, Praskovia Feodorovna announces that she has invited Mikhail Danilovitch, an ordinary doctor, to visit while the distinguished doctor is there so that he can discuss Ivan's condition with him. Danilovitch arrives at the appointed hour, and once again there are the tappings and listening and significant conversations about the kidney and blind gut in Ivan's presence and in the next room. All this nonsense, instead of the real question of life and death.

Doctor Leschititsky: Don't worry, Ivan Ilyich, we will pounce on these conditions and force them to behave.

Ivan Ilyich: (*timidly, yet hopeful*) Is there any chance of recovery?

Doctor Leschititsky: One cannot promise anything, but there is a possibility. Goodbye for now.

Scene 7

Narrator: Praskovia returns late that night after attending the theater with the rest of the family, and enters Ivan's room.

Praskovia: I think Gerasim should leave now. I would like to sit with you myself.

Ivan Ilyich: No. Go.

Praskovia: Are you suffering a lot?

Ivan Ilyich: It doesn't matter.

Praskovia: Take some opium.

Narrator: Ivan consented and drank it. Praskovia went away. Ivan was in an oppressive state of unconsciousness till three in the morning. It seemed to him that he and his pain were being pushed deeper and deeper into a long, narrow, black hole, yet couldn't be pushed right through. It was agonizing. He was afraid, yet wanted to fall through. He struggled against it, yet tried to help. Suddenly, he tore free and fell and came to. There he was, lying with his emaciated stockinged feet resting on Gerasim's shoulders. There was the same interminable pain.

Ivan Ilyich: Go away, Gerasim.

Gerasim: It doesn't matter. I'll sit a while.

Ivan Ilyich: No, do go.

Narrator: Gerasim left and then without constraint Ivan cried like a child. He cried for his helplessness, his terrible loneliness, people's cruelty, God's cruelty, and the absence of God.

Ivan Ilyich: God, why have You done all this? Why did You bring me here? What have I done that You torment me so dreadfully? But I know You will not answer. Go on, batter me! But what for? What have I done to You? What is it for?

Narrator: Then Ivan stopped crying and grew quiet as though he were listening not to a voice speaking to him, but to the voice of his own soul.

Ivan Ilyich: You ask me what I want. What do I need? Not to suffer. To live. Live how, you ask? Live like I did before. Pleasantly.

There was something good for me as a child, but that person is no more. Then, in law school there was something genuinely good there – enjoyment, friendship, hopes.

There were good moments in my Governor's service, and I remember love for women. As I think on through my life, there is less and less good. My marriage – at first so happy, then disillusion. The hypocrisy, the anxieties about money all those 20 years.

So what is this? What is it for? Surely it can't be that my life was so pointless, so wrong? And if it was that wrong and that pointless, then why die and die in pain? Something's not right here.

Maybe I didn't live as I should? But how could that be, when I did everything as I should have done? I want to live as I lived in court. Here he comes, the judge. But I'm not to blame. What is my guilt? Why this misery?

Scene 8

Narrator: Two weeks passed and Ivan Ilyich did not rise from his divan, lying nearly all the time with his face to the wall. He suffered alone. From the beginning of his illness, his life seemed split into two opposing and alternating moods – either despair and the expectation of incomprehensible and terrible death, or hope and the absorbing scrutiny of his bodily functions – his kidney or his gut. He existed now in a loneliness which could not have been more complete. His memories always began with the most recent in time and led back to the most distant, to his childhood, and there they stopped. The further back he went, the more life there was, the more kindness.

Ivan Ilyich: Just as my suffering grows worse and worse now, so the whole of my life went worse and worse. If only I could understand what it is for. It could only be explained if one could say I hadn't lived as I should. But to accept that would be quite impossible. There is no explanation! Suffering. Death. For what?

Narrator: The next two weeks passed in this way. One evening, Feodor Petrovitch made a formal proposal to marry Ivan's daughter. That same night, Ivan suffered another change for the worse. When Praskovia and Ivan's daughter, Liza, went into his room to tell him about the proposal, Ivan was moaning and staring fixedly in front of him. Praskovia started talking about medicines. But she stopped suddenly when he shifted his gaze to her and she saw the terrible look of hatred he had for her.

Ivan Ilyich: For the love of Christ, let me die in peace! You will both soon be free of me.

Narrator: Both women fell silent, sat a while, and then left the room.

Liza: (*whining*) It's just as though we were doing it *to* him! I'm sorry for Papa, but why should we be made miserable?

Narrator: Doctor Nikolaef arrived soon and Ivan answered his tiresome questions.

Ivan Ilyich: You know perfectly well you can do nothing, so leave it alone. You cannot even alleviate my suffering. Leave it!

Narrator: The doctor left the room and informed Praskovia that things were very bad and only opium could relieve the pain.

Doctor Nikolaef: His physical suffering is intense, but his moral suffering is worse, and that is what torments him most of all.

Narrator: Ivan's spiritual suffering had come suddenly during the night as he looked at Gerasim's kind, sleepy face with its high cheekbones. It was then Ivan questioned his life.

Ivan Ilyich: What if in reality the whole of my life was not done right? Could it be true that I have lived my whole life not as I should have done? It occurs to me that I never did fight against what people in high positions deemed good when they were wrong … I shrugged it off. And my work and the construction of my life and my family and my social and professional interests – all of them might be not the right thing. And if this is so, and I am leaving life in the knowledge that I have ruined everything that was given to me and it can't be put right, then what?

Praskovia: Ivan, sweetest, take the sacrament, do this for me. It can't do any harm and it often helps.

Ivan Ilyich: What? Take the sacrament? What for? There's no need. And yet –

Praskovia: Will you, my dear? I'll send for our priest, he's so nice.

Ivan Ilyich: Very well.

Narrator: When the priest heard his confession, Ivan felt a kind of ease from his doubts and his sufferings, and a moment's hope came to him. He started thinking again about his blind gut and the possibility of putting it right. He took the sacrament with tears in his eyes. His hope of life rose again.

Ivan Ilyich: (*quietly, to himself*) To live, I want to live!

Praskovia: It's true, isn't it? You're better.

Ivan Ilyich: Yes.

Narrator: As he looked at Praskovia, her clothes, the way she was put together, the expression on her face, the sound of her voice, it all said one thing to him. It was true, everything he had once lived by was a lie. And as soon as he thought that, the suffering returned, and with it the knowledge of inevitable, imminent death.

Ivan Ilyich: Go away! Get out! Let me be!

Scene 9

Narrator: From that minute began the three days of unremitting screaming, so dreadful with horror it could be heard beyond two closed doors.

Ivan Ilyich: I am lost. There is no return. The end has come, the very end. No!!!
I am being thrust into the black hole! I am unable to crawl into it for myself. It is because my life has been bad, that is the reason I cannot crawl into the hole. Let me go! Let me get into the hole, do not hold me tight. Why do you torment me?

Narrator: Now it is the third day, an hour before Ivan's death. Just then the little schoolboy, his son, Vassili, creeps into his father's room and comes up to his bed. The dying man is still screaming desperately and throwing his arms about. His hand falls on Vassili's head. The boy catches hold of it, presses it to his lips and bursts into tears.
It is just at this point that Ivan Ilyich falls through the hole, sees the glimmer of light and it becomes clear to him that his life has not been what it should have been, but that it could still be put right.

Ivan Ilyich: What is it I feel? Someone is kissing my hand.

Narrator: He opens his eyes and looks at his son. He feels sorrow for him. His wife comes into the room and he glances at her. She is gazing at him with a look of despair, her mouth open, tears on her nose and cheeks. He feels sorry for her. Too weak to speak, Ivan thinks, "Yes, I am making them miserable. They're sorry for me, but it will be better for them when I'm dead."

Ivan Ilyich: Take my son out. Sorry for him. Sorry for you. ... Propusti.

Narrator: He had wanted to say "Prosti – forgive me", but he said "Propusti – let me pass." Lacking the strength to correct himself, he gave up, knowing that the one who needed to know would understand him. Suddenly it became clear that what had been tormenting him was suddenly leaving him, falling away on all sides. He was sorry for them, he had to free them and free himself from all this pain.

Ivan Ilyich: How good and how simple. And where has the pain gone? Come on, where are you, pain? Yes, there it is. Well, never mind, let it be. And death? Where is it? But, where is my fear of death? I cannot find it. There is no death. Instead of death there is only light! What joy!!

Narrator: For him it all happened in a moment. For those around him, his agony continued for two hours. Gradually the snoring gurgle came less frequently. "It is finished" someone above him said.

Ivan Ilyich: Death is finished. There is no more death.

Narrator: He drew the air into himself, stopped in mid-breath, stretched, and died.

DISCUSSION QUESTIONS

1. What were your feelings as you read through the story? Did any of your feelings change over the course of the play?
2. How do members of Ivan's family relate to his illness? What are your feelings about Ivan himself, Ivan's colleagues, Praskovia, Ivan's son Vassili, Ivan's daughter Liza, and the physicians?
3. Who in the story needs to be cared for? Who is the primary caregiver and what is the role of this individual in Ivan's life?
4. How would you care for Ivan? What might you carry from this play into your own caring for others?
5. What do think is the meaning of the "black hole"?
6. What do you think about the ending of the story?
7. Do you think Tolstoy's existential concerns and his fear of death influenced his writing? If so, how?
8. Write one or two questions that you would ask about the play.

REFERENCE

Doyle NH, translator. *The Death of Ivan Ilyich*. New York: Crowell & Company; 1887.

REFLECTIONS ON THIS UNIT

Journal Note for Unit 1.1

____

____

____

____

ASSIGNMENT

Write your responses to the questions on the lines under **Exercise A *Relating to Death*** in Unit 2.1, and be prepared to discuss them in the next session.

REFERENCE

1. Quill T. *Caring for Patients at the End of Life*. Oxford: Oxford University Press; 2001.

Part 2:
Understanding the Caregiver's Self

The most important quality that we bring to caring for the dying is our own understanding of and relationship with dying and death. We all have inherited legacies from family and culture about the meaning of dying and death. To serve the dying, we need to understand these inherited legacies, and we need to confront our attitudes, fears, and any unfinished business that we have with past experiences. This kind of self-knowledge enhances in us the virtues of honesty, openness, and steadfastness. These qualities are frequently sensed and felt to be comforting by the dying. This kind of self-knowledge also provides the ground for giving to and receiving from another person. To keep company with the dying teaches us about the fragility of our own life and prepares us for our dying journey.

The Units in this Part provide an opportunity to better understand yourself as a person with deeply held attitudes, beliefs, and values, to examine your ideas about the meaning of death, to begin developing the skills of mindful presence and listening, and to explore your own sense of spirituality.

Unit 2.1: Reflecting on Death

KEY ISSUES

Awareness of death, ways of dying, imagining another's lifeworld, life and death needs and wishes.

(10 minutes) Quieting Exercise

The trainer will lead this exercise. Arrange your chair so that there is some distance between you and a table or others around you. Sit erect but not rigidly. Close your eyes. Breathe in as deeply as you can and force the breath back out as strongly as you can. Do this three times. Then just allow the breath to return to normal and let all of your thoughts go. Just sit in peace and silence for two minutes, and feel your breath as it moves across your nostrils. When you are ready, return to the room and sit quietly for a few moments before speaking.

(10 minutes) Journal Note Share

> *Our life is a journey that begins with birth and ends with death, and once we begin that journey, we are on our way, non-stop. There are no breathers, no time-outs. It is a one-shot deal. So we should relate to our life now, while we still can – but to do so, we must also learn to relate to our death.*
>
> Judith L. Lief (1:5)

INTRODUCTION

The phrase "sharing the journey with a dying person" conjures up wonderful images of selflessness and altruism, and while it truly is these things, it can be many other things as well. It can be humbling, fulfilling and gratifying, it can be demanding and confusing, and it can produce anxiety. Regardless of the kind of caregiver you are – professional, relative or friend, or volunteer – you will find that caring for a dying person will often bring out the very best in you, and that at other times you will find yourself sorely lacking in some way. How can you prepare for this compelling experience? Let us take our cue from Lief's words in the above quote – that it is critical to relate to death now, and to accept the fact that we are indeed on our own final path. At a later time, we shall consider in greater depth our own beliefs and feelings about death. For now, you will begin by recalling the death of a friend or loved one, how they died and how it affected you. Then you will consider what it meant to walk beside Ivan Ilyich on his journey, how he faced his dying time, and what could have made his journey easier. You will consider what you foresee your needs will be for your own time of dying, and finally you will consider what you as a caregiver will take into the relationship with a dying person and where and when you must observe boundaries to your caregiving.

EXERCISES

A. (15 minutes) *Relating to Death*

This exercise was assigned at the end of Unit 1.1. Write your responses to the following questions on the lines below. Share some of your responses with the large group.

How old were you when you first became aware of death? Was it the death of a person or a pet?

____

____

____

____

____

Were you present at the time of the death? If not, how did you hear about the death? How did you feel about it? How did you handle it?

____

____

____

B. (25 minutes) *Ways of Dying*

Some individuals die peacefully and gracefully, while others suffer with fear and anxiety. You may have experienced the death of a loved one or friend. Describe to the large group how that experience was for the dying person and how it was for you. Recall how Ivan Ilyich experienced dying.

C. (45 minutes) *Moral Imagination Exercise*

Turn back to Unit 1.1, *The Death of Ivan Ilyich*, and for three or four minutes scan through the play to reacquaint yourself with the characters and the story. Choose *one* of the following characters: Ivan, Praskovia, Liza, Vassili, or Gerasim. *In the voice of that character*, write on the lines below how they feel about their place in Ivan's life and death story. Your writing can be in the form of a short essay, a poem, a journal entry, or a letter. Do not feel uncomfortable or worried about your writing ability, just write. Write as neatly and clearly as possible.

You are encouraged to share your writing with the group. Before you read your composition, tell the group what character you chose and how you felt being that person.

If several people have written about the same character, everyone in that group should read their pieces before moving on to another character. This enables you to observe how perceptions about the same person or circumstance differ, and provides you with the opportunity to get to know your fellow classmates better. Questions may be asked about another person's writing for clarification, but not to challenge their thinking or reasoning.

Name of the character you chose:____

D. (45 minutes) *The Needs of the Dying*

For the first 5 minutes, reflect on the needs you will have in your time of dying. Write your responses on the following lines. Form dyads or small groups of three or four and share your responses.

Next, in your small group, discuss and write responses to the following questions:

- What do you believe are the needs of individuals who are in the dying process?
- What did your relative or friend need?
- What did Ivan Ilyich need to make his journey easier?

Write your small group responses on the lines below, and then share your responses with the large group. As the large group works on this exercise, list the various needs on the blackboard or chart paper. For future reference and editing, copy this list on the lines provided below.

Needs of the Dying Chart

Empty handed I entered the world
Barefoot I leave it.
My coming, my going –
Two simple happenings
That got entangled.
Kozan Ichikyo (2: 108)

(5 MINUTES) REFLECTIONS ON THIS UNIT

Journal Note for Unit 2.1

ASSIGNMENT

(To be determined by the trainer.)

ADDITIONAL RESOURCES

1. Colby WH. *Long Goodbye: the deaths of Nancy Cruzan*. Carlsbad, CA: Hay House, Inc.; 2007.
2. Kubler-Ross E. *On Death and Dying*. New York: Scribner Classics; 1969.

Three books are particularly helpful for exploring further how you relate to death. Each contains several meditation exercises that you can practice.

1. Halifax J. *Being With Dying: cultivating compassion and fearlessness in the presence of death*. Boston, MA: Shambhala; 2008.
2. Lief J. *Making Friends With Death: a Buddhist guide to encountering mortality*. Boston, MA: Shambhala; 2001.
3. Longaker C. *Facing Death and Finding Hope: a guide to the emotional and spiritual care of the dying*. London: Century; 1997.

REFERENCES

1. Lief JL. *Making Friends With Death: a Buddhist guide to encountering mortality*. Boston, MA: Shambhala; 2001.
2. Hoffman Y. *Japanese Death Poems*. Boston, MA: Tuttle Publishing; 1986.

Unit 2.2: Mindfulness

KEY ISSUES

Mindfulness, presence, mindful listening, meditation.

(10 minutes) Quieting Exercise (see Unit 2.1)

(10 minutes) Journal Note Share

> *Whatever we call it – "mindfulness", "bodyfulness", "soulfulness", or "heartfulness" – meditation has to do with bringing our body, our thoughts and emotions and our breath into harmony.*
>
> Judith Lief (1: 55)

INTRODUCTION

Two skills that are central to caregiving are the ability to attend fully to the dying person and to listen carefully. These two skills engender trust and openness in the relationship, they enable the dying person to share their innermost thoughts, and they lay the groundwork for compassionate care. The focus of this Unit will be on these two essential skills, which we more formally call "mindful presence and mindful listening." You might respond, "Well, of course, if I visit the dying person, I'm there, I'm present, and of course I would listen." However, there is much more to these two skills than is at first apparent. Jon Kabat-Zinn (2: 108,109) speaks of being mindful in the following way:

> Mindfulness can be thought of as a moment-to-moment, non-judgmental awareness, cultivated by paying attention in a specific way, that is, in the present moment, and as non-reactively, as non-judgmentally, and as open-heartedly as possible. ... Mindfulness is none other than the capacity we all already have to know what is happening as is it is happening. ... For most of us, it *has* to be refined through practice.

Throughout this program, when we speak of mindful presence and mindful listening, the words of Kabat-Zinn serve as our framework. It means that we put aside our own concerns and agenda and bestow our entire attention, in a relaxed yet observant manner, to the other. It means perceiving the physical and emotional state and the *spirit* of the other person and, with words or in silence, responding supportively. Being mindfully present with another is perhaps the greatest gift we can give – being there quietly with our heart and soul open, with body, emotions, and thoughts stilled, denying our desire to interject, implore, or impugn, and knowing that silence will provide the quiet and necessary space for the other to touch his own soul. (Interesting note: *listen* contains the same letters as *silent.)*

Why are you so afraid of silence?
Silence is the root of everything.
If you spiral into its void
a hundred voices will thunder messages
you so long to hear.

Rumi (3: 11)

Mindfulness can best be nurtured through the regular practice of meditation. Basic meditation has two complementary dimensions: mindfulness and awareness. In our everyday lives, our minds are restless, always jumping from one thing to another. It is difficult to pay attention under these circumstances. So we need to quiet the mind – be mindful – so that we can experience and practice relaxed awareness (1,2).

Although many people are at first reluctant to engage in meditation, seeing it as somewhat mystical and belonging only to certain religious or cultural groups, in reality everyone meditates – only the form or focus of meditation differs. Even such things as sitting quietly and focusing on the waves as they gently break on the shore, following the movement of the soft wind as it wafts across a field of grain, focusing on colorful leaves as they dance in the breeze, or listening mindfully to soothing music are simple forms of meditation. The meditation that we introduce in this Unit is a practiced, intentional form. Additional forms such as visualization, guided imagery, body scan, gradual stress relaxation, and moving meditations that include yoga, tai chi, and mindful walking are also beneficial. Allthough the methods and practices are countless, they are all directed toward the same goal – to calm the mind, body and spirit and become mindful in the present moment.

There is increasing evidence that practicing meditation can effectively reduce stress and anxiety, improve emotional and physical health and the ability to deal with illness, enhance overall life enjoyment, and increase empathy for others. In view of these many benefits, you can see why practicing meditation can greatly benefit the dying person as well as the caregiver. Christine Longaker (4: 64), author of *Facing Death and Finding Hope*, writes:

> The real meaning of "meditation" is to sustain the flow of pure awareness, free of duality – pure, simple, naked presence – an awareness without commentary or reactions, a pure presence of profound peace and unbiased love, free of grasping after external things and free of our sense of "self" the "grasper." And this is the ultimate relief from suffering – dissolving our habitual identification with the selfish ego and arriving at the profound peace and bliss of our true nature.

In this Unit you will first practice a basic "quieting" or "sitting" meditation, and then you will practice two simple mindful presence exercises. Before visiting a dying person, the caregiver should find a quiet place to "sit" for a few moments in order to settle the mind and become grounded.

EXERCISES

A. (40 minutes) *Mindfulness Meditation: Quieting Exercise or Sitting*

The practice of mindfulness meditation helps us to develop our capacity to focus, direct, and maintain our attention. It enables us to concentrate our energy on what we are experiencing. Through mindfulness, we develop our composure and an increased sensitivity to both verbal and nonverbal communication. The regular practice of mindfulness meditation will help the caregiver to listen mindfully to the dying person and discern his or her feelings as well as their own. Let us practice two types of mindfulness meditation now. Your trainer will lead you in these exercises.

The most fundamental way of developing the capacities noted above is to begin by focusing on your breath and allowing it to become the anchor of your mind. You may sit in a chair, lie on your back on the floor, or sit on a pillow on the floor with your legs crossed at the ankles, or in the lotus position. If you use a chair, it may be a straight chair or have arms. Position your chair so that you are away from any other object or person. Relax and sit squarely and comfortably and feel your chair supporting you with your spine erect but not rigid. (Kabat-Zinn describes this as "sitting with dignity.") Place both feet flat on the floor and allow your hands to rest on the chair arms or on the tops of your thighs or gently in your lap with your fingers loose. If you sit on the floor, let your arms lie comfortably beside you. Close your eyes. If this is not comfortable, then find a spot somewhere toward the floor out in front of you and allow your eyes to lose focus. Breathe in as deeply as possible and then push the breath out forcibly through your mouth, even making a "whooshing" sound as the air moves out. Repeat this cleansing breath three times.

Now allow your breath to return to its natural rhythm, and try to reach into the center of your being. Feel your breath as it moves in and out of your nostrils. Do not force your breath – just allow it to move naturally in and out. Consciously move the breath down below your diaphragm and feel your abdomen rise and fall with each breath. Continue with this quiet "belly-breathing", paying attention to each breath. If a thought comes into your head, recognize it, do not argue with it or judge it or push it away, just gently let it go and return to your breath. If you hear a noise or disturbance within or outside the room, acknowledge it and then just gently let it go and return to your breath. Between your out-breath and your next in-breath, feel the absolute peace and quiet in your body and mind. Continue with your breathing for several more minutes.

When you are ready, slowly return your consciousness to the room. When you have fully returned and before you discuss the experience, sit quietly and think about what you experienced and how you felt during this meditation. If you were unable to do this quieting exercise, practice it again later, always paying attention to the breath. Be patient and eventually you will be able to do it.

In the second meditation, begin with the sitting exercise you just learned in the first meditation above. When you become still and centered, allow your focus to shift to one comfortable sound in the room where you are right now – maybe the hum of a motor or the ticking of a clock. Let this comfortable sound be the anchor for your focus. As other thoughts, noises, or feelings intrude, acknowledge them and gently let them go. Continue in this way until you are ready to return to this room. Before speaking, sit quietly and think about what you experienced and how you felt during this meditation.

B. (45 minutes) *Being Mindfully Present*

Once you have quieted yourself, it is easier to be present to one another, simply sitting still without any pretense. This quiet and attentive state can provide a great deal of comfort to both you and the dying person. Form dyads and sit facing your partner. Your trainer will lead you through this exercise.

Close your eyes and, for the next 2 minutes, pay attention to your breath and find that silent place at your center. Become acutely aware of your inner being – be present to yourself. What are you thinking? What are you feeling? What are you experiencing? Become aware of your own spiritual being.

Now open your eyes and in the next few moments, without exchanging any words, become aware of your partner. What do you see in them? What do you feel? What do you experience in them? Try to feel their spirit. Do not speak – just be present and aware in silence with the other.

On the lines below, write a few words to describe how it felt to be present to yourself and then how it felt to be present to your partner. Share your thoughts with your partner. Share some of your thoughts with the entire group.

There is a channel between voice and presence,
a way where information flows.
In disciplined silence the channel opens,
in wandering talk, it closes.

Rumi (3: 25)

C. (45 minutes) *Listening Mindfully to the Other's Story*

For this exercise you will once again work in pairs. You may change your partner or keep the same one that you had for the preceding exercise. Decide which one of you will be the first to tell a story. The story should be only 5 minutes in length, and should deal with an experience that had a considerable impact on your life. While the storyteller is considering what story to tell and how to tell it in 5 minutes, the listener should be "sitting" – quieting him- or herself and preparing to hear the other's story. When both are ready, the storyteller will begin. The listener will not interject, ask questions, or respond, but will simply be mindfully present. They will have good eye contact, nod their head when appropriate, perhaps reaching out and touching the other person – all to indicate to the storyteller that they are listening carefully. We acknowledge that because it is our human nature to respond to another's story, this exercise may feel artificial and awkward, but the ability to be silent is an important skill to learn and practice. At the end of the 5 minutes, when the story has finished, the storyteller will write on the lines below how it felt to be listened to mindfully in silence. The listener will write how it felt to listen mindfully without responding in any way. Then switch roles and repeat the exercise. When you have completed the exercise, share what you wrote with your partner, and then share in the large group.

(15 MINUTES) REFLECTIONS ON THIS UNIT

Journal Note for Unit 2.2

ASSIGNMENT

Practice the sitting meditation each day for 10–15 minutes. Share your experience in the next session.

ADDITIONAL RESOURCES

There are numerous excellent audio materials and books that guide you through various meditations. We have found the following helpful:

1. Kabat-Zinn J. *Guided Mindfulness Meditation: Series 1, Series 2, Series 3.* These may be obtained at www.mindfulnesstapes.com
2. Kornfield J. *Guided Meditation: six essential practices to cultivate love, awareness, and wisdom.* These CDs may be obtained at www.soundstrue.com
3. Kornfield J. *Meditation for Beginners: six meditations for insight, inner clarity, and cultivating a compassionate heart.* Boulder, CO: Sounds True; 2004.
4. Nhat Hanh T. *The Miracle of Mindfulness: a manual on meditation.* Boston, MA: Beacon Press; 1975.
5. Nhat Hanh T. *The Blooming of a Lotus: guided meditation for achieving the miracle of mindfulness.* Boston, MA: Beacon Press; 1993.
6. Santorelli S. *Heal Thy Self: lessons on mindfulness in medicine.* New York: Bell Tower; 1999.
7. Wilson JL. When words aren't enough. *Lutheran Partners.* 2000; **March/April:** 53–4.
8. Kabat-Zinn J. *Guided Mindfulness Meditation Series I.* Stress reduction tapes and CDs. PO Box 547, Lexington, MA 024230.
9. Nhat Hanh T. *Plum Village Meditations.* 1997. Sounds True, PO Box 8010, Dept B, Boulder, CO 80306.
10. Voces Novae. *Meditations on Life and Death.* PO Box 802, Clear Creek, IN 47426.

11. Levine S, Levine O. *The Grief Process: meditations for healing*. 1999. Sounds True, PO Box 8010, Dept B, Boulder, CO 80306.

REFERENCES

1. Lief JL. *Making Friends With Death: a Buddhist guide to encountering mortality*. Boston, MA: Shambhala; 2001.
2. Kabat-Zinn J. *Coming to Our Senses: healing ourselves and the world through mindfulness.* New York: Hyperion; 2005.
3. Kolin AM, Mafi M, translators. *Rumi: hidden music*. London: Thorsons/HarperCollins Publisher; 2001.
4. Longaker C. *Facing Death and Finding Hope: a guide to the emotional and spiritual care of the dying*. London: Century; 1997.

Unit 2.3: Self-Knowledge

KEY ISSUES

Personhood, self-awareness, self-knowledge, caregiver attributes and motives.

(10 minutes) Sitting Meditation

(10 minutes) Share meditation practice experience as assigned in Unit 2.2

(10 minutes) Journal Share

> *If people are to grow, if they are to move toward authenticity and reach their potential, then they must identify those feelings and issues that control them. Otherwise those feelings and issues imprison and ultimately define them.*
>
> Stephen P. Kliewer and John Saultz (1: 111)

INTRODUCTION

The human being is a complex integration of four elements, namely the physical being (the body), the psychological being (the self that holds our thoughts and feelings), the social being (the self that relates to our various environments and the others in our lives) and the spiritual being (the self that embraces our beliefs about human existence – for example, *I am an integral part of nature*). The interconnectedness of these four beings creates the unique and dynamic personhood that each of us possesses.

Before attending to a dying person, caregivers must first examine and attend to their own personhood, ensuring that all four "beings" are healthy and intact and ready to assume the work of caregiving – the bedside is certainly not the place or the time to heal one's own wounds or bruises. It is essential that caregivers understand the effect that their own beliefs and emotional state may have on the dying person, and identify those times when they do not have the steadiness of mind or heart to attend to the other. On this matter, Mark Nepo (2: 30), philosopher, poet, and cancer survivor, has written:

> It is said that those who are in pain can no longer fear pain, just as those who are in water can no longer stay dry. Instead, they fear drowning. And just as one who soothes another's loneliness is made less lonely, those tired angels who accept another's pain are made more whole by this acceptance. ... And those still wet with pain know they cannot be healed by anyone whose emptiness is greater than their own.

Becoming and remaining aware of the self enables us to question our feelings and attitudes and to understand the rules and forces that shape us, control us, and define us. It requires significant practice, and the more we practice it the better we become at it. Only with self-knowledge can we work to change negative attitudes and behaviors, strengthen our weaknesses, and move forward. As we attend to the dying person it is not enough that we are acutely aware of the other, noting their reactions and responses; in the same moment we need to observe and monitor our own reactions and responses. In this Unit we shall practice exercises to increase our self-awareness and self-knowledge.

EXERCISES

A. (50 minutes) *Self-Knowledge*

For the first 15 minutes, write responses to each of the questions across all of the exercises in section A. Share your responses with a partner, and then share with the large group.

1. Your Four Beings

Let us consider the four components of your total being – physical, psychological, social, and spiritual. Write a brief statement about each of your four "beings." For each element indicate whether it is intact and healthy, whether there are broken and painful areas. If you find wounds or bruises, what causes them? How might this condition affect your caregiving?

Your physical being:

____

____

____

Your psychological being:

Your social being:

Your spiritual being:

2. Your Personal Qualities

What personal qualities do you possess that you are particularly proud of?

Choose the one which you believe makes the strongest and clearest statement about who you are. When does this quality generally come into action?

How do you feel when this quality is in action?

How might this quality affect your caregiving?

Now list the qualities that you are least proud of.

Choose the one you least like in yourself. When does this quality come into action?

How do you feel when this quality is in action?

Which of your least favorable qualities is likely to "switch on" when you feel overstressed, challenged, or frustrated?

What steps might you take to minimize the possibility of such a "switching on"?

How might this personal quality affect your caregiving?

Do you want to change this quality? If so, how will you proceed? When will you begin?

3. Personal Control

List the times when you felt you were not in control of what was happening to you. How did you feel? How did you react? What resulted from your reactions?

Why might a dying person feel "out of control"? How might this feeling affect the dying person?

Did Ivan Ilyich feel "out of control"? In what way?

4. Emotional Pain

Think about times when you have recently felt emotional pain. What was your reaction to the pain? Did you blame something or someone else for the pain? Do you still have these feelings?

Why might a dying person feel emotional pain? How might this affect the person?

B. (50 minutes) *Caregiver Attributes*

Form groups of three or four and discuss the following question:

What knowledge, skills, attitudes, and behaviors do you believe are important for a caregiver to possess?

With a marker pen write the group responses on chart paper and mount the paper on a nearby wall for everyone to see. Compare and discuss the responses from all of the groups. You will find that some items will be duplicated and can be eliminated. Now construct a *Caregiver Attributes Chart* that best represents the characteristics on which everyone agrees. Copy the chart onto the lines below. As you continue to learn about caregiving, you can edit and/or expand this chart.

Caregiver Attributes Chart

____

____

____

____

____

____

____

____

C. (30 minutes) *Sharing the Journey*

For the first 10 minutes, write responses to all of the questions. Then share them with the large group.

Why do you want to share the journey with a dying person?

____

____

____

____

Do you possess the necessary qualities? What are these?

____

____

____

What do you need to learn?

____

____

____

How do you want to change?

____

____

____

How can you achieve the changes you desire? When will you begin?

____

____

____

How did you feel as you worked on the exercises in this Unit?

____

____

____

What did you learn about yourself by doing the exercises in this Unit?

____

____

____

Were you surprised by some of your responses or by something that you learned?

____

____

____

(5 MINUTES) REFLECTIONS ON THIS UNIT

Journal Note for Unit 2.3

____

____

____

____

____

____

ASSIGNMENT

For the next session, read the following poem by Rumi very carefully, and then write your interpretation on the lines below.

The Guest House
This being human is a guest house.
Every morning a new arrival
A joy, a depression, a meanness,
some momentary awareness comes
as an unexpected visitor.
Welcome and entertain them all!
Even if they are a crowd of sorrows,
who violently sweep your house
empty of all its furniture,
still, treat each guest honorably.
He may be clearing you out
for some new delight.
The dark thought, the shame, the malice,
meet them at the door laughing
and invite them in.
Be grateful for whatever comes,
because each has been sent
as a guide from beyond.
Rumi (3: 109)

REFERENCES

1. Kliewer SP, Saultz J. *Healthcare and Spirituality*. Oxford: Radcliffe Publishing; 2006.
2. Nepo M. Falling off and beginning again. In: *Proceedings of the Eighth Humanism and the Healing Arts Conference*, Institute for Professionalism Inquiry, Summa Health System; Akron, Ohio; 2008: 30–36.
3. Kolin AM, Mafi M, translators. *Rumi: hidden music*. London: Thorsons/HarperCollins Publisher; 2001.

Unit 2.4: Spiritual Knowledge

KEY ISSUES

Personhood, spirituality, relationship between spirituality and religion, presence.

(10 minutes) Meditation

(10 minutes) Journal Note Share

(10 minutes) Interpretations of the Rumi poem as assigned in Unit 2.3

> *Our spirituality is therefore the very roots of our being – who we think we are, why we are here and what we should do with our lives.*
>
> Stephen G. Wright (1: 77)

INTRODUCTION

As we discussed earlier, the human being is a complex integration of four unique components, namely the physical being, the psychological being, the social being, and the spiritual being. For heuristic purposes, we have separated personhood into four elements in order to envision the nature of each. However, as we have noted, they are intricately linked, each integrated with and influencing the others, and they are indivisible. In Unit 2.3 you briefly examined each of these components of your personhood and then focused in particular on your psychological being. It is not difficult to see the physical aspects of an individual – their body – and we can observe the behaviors that we attribute to the psychological and social beings. However, although we often attempt to relate certain qualities of an individual to the spiritual being, this entity tends to remain quite obscure. For this reason we shall, in this Unit, focus on the spiritual aspect in order to understand better how our spiritual being influences our personhood. Wendy Greenstreet (2: 9) conceptualizes the integration of the spiritual, physical–spiritual, social–spiritual, and psychological–spiritual components of being a person in the following diagram:

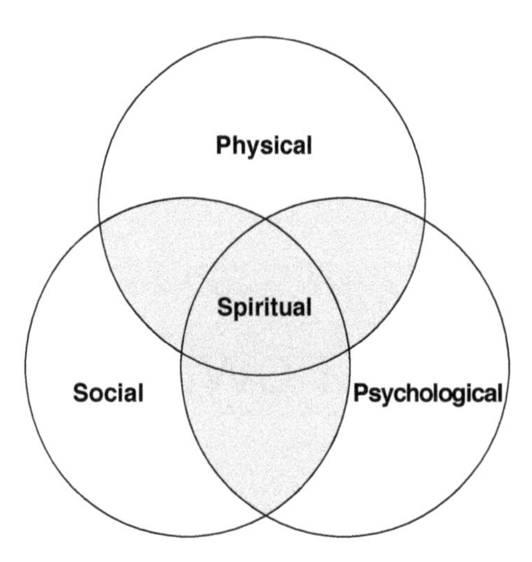

Figure 1: Spiritual, physical–spiritual, social–spiritual, and psychological–spiritual components of being a person.

About the spiritual being, Greenstreet (2: 9) writes:

> Each person has a spiritual dimension that may be expressed in religion, existential meaning, through relationships, and in hope and forgiveness as part of "becoming." The boundaries of the concept of spirituality are murky and its core is difficult to define, but its relation to "humanness" and humanity's relation to the universe are fundamentals.

Although there are features common to the various conceptions of spirituality, we each have our own construct. To a large degree, this construct is part of the framework for how we live.

In end-of-life care, spiritual issues can become monumental. Some dying persons find peace and hope as they draw near to death, while others may struggle with their situation and experience considerable spiritual anguish. *Why me? Why now? Who will care for my loved ones? What comes after death?* The caregiver should be prepared to hear these questions, acknowledge their importance and commonness, and discuss them sensitively. In Unit 2.3 we emphasized the need to practice continually self-awareness for increased self-knowledge and personal improvement and stability. Likewise, frequent reflection on your own spiritual being and your own journey will aid your spiritual stability and enable you to interact more effectively with the dying person. Understanding your own spiritual nature and how you differ from others is essential.

In this Unit you will have the privilege of learning about the spiritual beliefs and practices of your colleagues. Being open and generous in your discussions and accepting of others' beliefs and values is critical.

EXERCISES

A. (60 minutes) *Defining Spirituality**

Let us begin by thinking about *spirituality* – what it means to you, what it means to others, and how it relates to religion. The following two exercises will help you to become aware of how people differ in the way they view spirituality and the role that it plays in their lives.

For the first 10 minutes write your responses to the questions below. Then form groups of three or four and compare responses. **Note:** People's answers may differ; each answer must be honored, not challenged. Appoint one person as reporter for your group. With a marker pen, write your group's answers on chart paper and mount it on a nearby wall for easy viewing by the entire group. Begin with the first question and compare answers from every small group. Then move on to the next question. When both questions have been discussed, attempt to construct a *working definition* of spirituality that you can refer to later. After the group definition has been determined, compare it with those of other authors provided at the end of this Unit.

How do you define spirituality?

____

____

____

____

____

____

Is there a difference between spirituality and religion? If so, what is it?

____

____

____

____

____

* Exercises A and B and Assignment 2 are adaptations of an exercise developed by Peter Ways and Lura Pethtel for a medical student workshop.

B. (30 minutes) *Spirituality and Religion: Visualizing the Relationship*

A Venn diagram is a figure, usually composed of circles, that is used to show the relationship between two or more ideas or domains. Here we shall use two circles, one to represent spirituality (S) and the other to represent religion (R). The amount of overlap between the two circles indicates the degree of common relationship or what they share in common. The figures can vary from no overlap, indicating no shared relationship between the two ideas, to complete overlap, indicating that the two ideas are the same in all important ways. Study the following diagrams that represent how closely spirituality and religion are related for three individuals – Mary, Tom and Frank. How do you interpret each diagram?

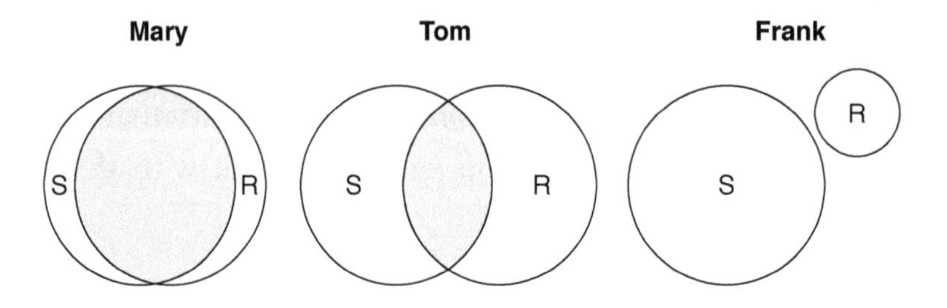

After the large group discussion of the diagrams, on another piece of paper or on the chalkboard draw a Venn diagram that represents how you relate spirituality and religion for yourself. Draw it large enough for others in the group to see. Share your diagram with the group. Copy your diagram in the space below or attach it in this section.

C. (30 minutes) *Large Group Discussion*

1. Was there a time in your life when you felt the presence of something – a spiritual presence or energy? Describe the experience, its source, and how you related to it (e.g. fear, anxiety, ecstasy, indifference).

2. When you look at a person or get to know them well, what is it about that person that might cause you to think "That person is spiritual"?
3. How do you regenerate or renew your spirit?

(5 MINUTES) REFLECTIONS ON THIS UNIT

JOURNAL NOTE FOR UNIT 2.4

____

____

____

____

____

ASSIGNMENT*

For the next session, see Exercise A, Unit 2.5. Create a model that represents aspects of your spirituality. For example, you could (a) construct a model, (b) draw or paint a picture or poster, (c) create a collage of pictures/photographs, or (d) assemble a collection of items. You may use any materials, and you may include music, poetry, or other art forms to enhance your creation. This is **not** to be a prose writing that you read to the class, but rather an actual physical entity that you show to the class and then describe any meaning that you attribute to it. As you work on this assignment, think about the following issues:

- How do you define spirituality for yourself? Did this change for you as you worked on your model?
- What were the spiritual aspects of your early life?
- Have you grown spiritually? How?
- What are your spiritual practices?
- Have you experienced transcendent/sacred/holy events that have influenced the way you live or believe?
- Do your spiritual beliefs influence the way you think about your death or after-death?
- How would you like to be remembered after you die? What legacy do you want to leave?

* This exercise was designed by Lura Pethtel and Peter Ways for an earlier workshop.

- How do you refresh or regenerate your spirit?
- What goals do you want to accomplish before you die?

ADDITIONAL RESOURCES

The following books provide useful perspectives on the general topic of spirituality/religion and healthcare.

1. Kliewer SP, Saultz J. *Healthcare and Spirituality*. Oxford: Radcliffe Publishing; 2006.
2. Koenig HG. *Spirituality in Patient Care: why, how, when, and what*. Philadelphia, PA: Templeton Foundation Press; 2002.
3. Pellegrino ED, Thomasma DC. *Helping and Healing: religious commitment in health care*. Washington, D.C.: Georgetown University Press; 1997.
4. Ronaldson S, ed. *Spirituality: the heart of nursing*. Melbourne: Ausmed Publications; 1984.
5. Levine S. *A Gradual Awakening*. New York: Anchor Books; 1997.

REFERENCES

1. Wright SG. Soul works: the relevance of spirituality to a healthy workplace. In: W Greenstreet (ed.) *Integrating Spirituality in Health and Social Care: perspectives and practical approaches*. Oxford: Radcliffe Publishing; 2006; pp. 76–85.
2. Greenstreet W, ed. *Integrating Spirituality in Health and Social Care: perspectives and practical approaches*. Oxford: Radcliffe Publishing; 2006.

DEFINITIONS OF SPIRITUALITY

*The word **spiritual** is ambiguous. As I use it, **spiritual** refers to concerns about the ultimate meaning and values in life. It has to do with our deepest sense of who we are and what life is all about. **Spiritual** does not imply any belief in a supreme being or in a life after this. Atheists have spiritual concerns just like everyone else.*

John Hardwig (1: 28)

The spiritual dimension, then, is that aspect of the person concerned with meaning and the search for the absolute reality that underlies the world of the senses and the mind and, as such, is distinct from adherence to a religious system. We recognize it in the values we hold, our sense of greater purpose, the faith upon which our world-view and actions are based, and in moments of direct experience.

John F. Hiatt, M.D. (2: 737)

Spirituality may be thought of as that which gives meaning to life and draws one to transcendence, to whatever is larger than or goes beyond the limits of the individual human lifetime. Spirituality is a broader concept than religion. Other expressions of spirituality may include prayer, meditation, being in community with others, involvement with the natural world, or relationship with a transcendent reality. Religion may be one expression of spirituality, but certainly not all spiritual persons are religious.

Thomason and Brody (3: 96–7)

This spiritual dimension is the human capacity to interpret, integrate, focus, organize, and even transcend what the rest of the individual's capacities collectively experience.

Orr, Samarza, and Alexander (4: 26)

... a quality that goes beyond religious affiliation, that strives for inspirations, reverence, awe, meaning and purpose, even in those who do not believe in God. The spiritual dimension tries to be in harmony with the universe, strives for answers

about the infinite and comes into focus when the person faces emotional stress, physical illness and death.

Murray and Zentner (5: 259)

... spirituality is generally seen as experiential in nature. It has less to do with doctrines, ideas, or even rituals, and more to do with inner feelings, movement, or impact within the world of emotions, the realm of the heart. It is not that spirituality does not involve practices or ritual, but these activities tend to be more individualistic rather than organized or formal, and are geared at stimulating inner movement or growth.

Kliewer and Saultz (6: 73)

REFERENCES

1. Hardwig J. Spiritual issues at the end of life: a call for discussion. *Hastings Report.* 2000; **30:** 28–30.
2. Hiatt JD. *South Med J.* 1986; **79:** 736–43.
3. Thomason CL, Brody H. Inclusive spirituality. *J Fam Pract.* 1992; **48:** 96–7.
4. Orr RD, Samarza A, Alexander W. Integrative rounds: one approach to whole person care. *Ann Behav Sci Med Educ.* 1996; **3:** 22–31.
5. Murray RB, Zentner JB. *Nursing Concepts for Health Promotion.* London: Prentice Hall; 1989.
6. Kliewer SP, Saultz J. *Healthcare and Spirituality.* Oxford: Radcliffe Publishing; 2006.

Unit 2.5 The Whole Self: Body–Mind–Spirit

KEY ISSUES

Spiritual awareness, needs for life and death, goals for personal growth, body–mind–spirit integration, meditation, mindfulness.

(10 minutes) Meditation

(10 minutes) Journal Note Share

> *A great mystery of wellness centers on the effort to find and re-find our steady place in the Universal stream. What drains us, pulls us away from the stream. What sustains us, brings us back into that luminous stream.*
>
> Mark Nepo (1: 30)

INTRODUCTION

In Unit 2.4 we discovered how differently we view spirituality and how it affects our lives, and we also found commonalities in our viewpoints. Ways, Engel and Finkelstein (2: 181) have this to say about spirituality:

> Your *spirituality* manifests the best of yourself. It expresses the values and meanings without which you will founder. It involves the acquisition, expression, and honoring of those qualities, values, and behaviors that define the kind of person you want to be. It is, for most of us, the essence of our bond to other individuals, to family, to larger communities of friendship and service, and to a transcendent being or set of values.

In this Unit we shall continue our exploration of spirituality in greater depth through interviews and participants' *spiritual models*. and examine the linkages among the four facets of our personhood. You will recall Greenstreet's diagram which placed spirituality at the "core of the integrated whole." Although we don't often think about these linkages, they are regularly evident in our daily lives.

EXERCISES

A. (70 minutes) *Spiritual Models*

The assignment for this Unit requested that you create a model that represents aspects of your spirituality. Each trainee will have 5 to 8 minutes to present their spiritual model. Other trainees may ask questions to clarify, but not to challenge, the presenter's creation or the meaning for the presenter. In the large group, discuss how people differ in their spiritual beliefs and how these beliefs might influence their lives.

B. (40 minutes) *Reflection*

Form dyads. For 15 minutes share your thoughts about the following questions. Then share some of your thoughts with the large group.

- Did your definition of spirituality change as you worked on your model?
- What were the spiritual aspects of your early life?
- Have you grown spiritually? How?
- What did you learn about yourself as you constructed your spiritual model?
- What were some of the similarities you found in your beliefs to those of others in the group?
- How do you want to grow spiritually?
- How can you achieve the changes that you desire?

C. (30 minutes) *Body–Mind–Spirit Linkages*

Recall a time in your past when you suffered a loss – perhaps the death of a close friend or relative or a beloved pet, or maybe you lost your job or your wallet or your home, or possibly you were injured or became seriously ill and disabled for a period of time. During that experience did you suffer physically? Did you suffer psychologically? Did you suffer socially? Did you suffer spiritually? On the following lines, write a few brief notes about the event and the reactions that you experienced. Share these with a partner and then share some of your thoughts with the large group.

____

____

____

(5 MINUTES) REFLECTIONS ON THIS UNIT

Journal Note for Unit 2.5

ASSIGNMENT

(To be determined by the trainer.)

REFERENCES

1. Nepo M. Falling off and beginning again. In: *Proceedings of the Eighth Humanism and the Healing Arts Conference*, Summa Health System, Akron, OH; 2008: 30–36.
2. Ways P, Engel JD, Finkelstein P. *Clinical Clerkships: the heart of professional development*. Thousand Oaks, CA: Sage Publications; 2000.

Unit 2.6: Facing Death

KEY ISSUES

Dying is unknown territory, dying well, relating to death, terminal prognosis.

(10 minutes) Meditation

(10 minutes) Journal Note Share

> *As we go about our life, and especially in working with the sick and dying, we should never forget that we, too, are dying.*
>
> Judith Lief (1: 13)

INTRODUCTION

Too often death is depicted as a fearsome specter draped in black robes and carrying a scythe, ready to cut us down. For some, however, the conception is much more pleasant and welcoming. My (LLP) friend who lay for several years captive in a body crippled with disease begged for her dear friend, Death, to release her from her agony. My father saw Death as an old buddy, but was surprised when it came abruptly in the middle of the night to claim him. And, early one evening, my mother settled down peacefully upon her bed and welcomed Death as it gently enfolded her in its arms and quietly spirited her away. Our (LLP and JDE) dear friend, who was always telling stories and jokes, did so until his last breath. To the contrary, some others in our lives did not envision death as such an amiable visitor. Like most of us they were aware that death would come, but they refused to think about it or plan for it or prepare themselves emotionally, psychologically, or spiritually.

We know that millions upon millions of people die every year, yet we continue to try every way possible to avoid the subject. It is taboo; we don't even like to say the word. Instead, we use terms like "*he's passed away* (or *on* or *over)*", "*he's gone*", *or* "*he's in the great beyond.*" We often use jokes and laughter about death to lessen the power that it has on us and to shield us from the fear it engenders. The result of our evasive tactics is that the moment we learn that our illness or condition is terminal, we are thrust into a brand new landscape – an unknown territory – and we are not ready. Rather than shying away from thinking about death, let us take this opportunity right here, right now, to face death head on. Virginia Morris (2: 93,103) encourages us to "step even closer":

> We all know we are headed for a crash. We need to step closer and then even closer still, until we feel the cold gust of death upon our souls. This is the frigid inner sanctum, where death is personal and real. It is not an easy place to be, but neither is it as horrible as we imagine. ... Whatever your own fears and dreads and concerns are, tease them out one by one, examine them carefully, try to address them, and then revisit them at another time, for they will change.

Ideally, dying well means not suffering physical pain, but also maintaining control and self-direction, retaining self-esteem, completing relationships with grace, saying goodbye to loved ones, finding peace, and embracing eternity. Kathleen Dowling Singh (3: 1) speaks thoughtfully about this, as she writes:

> The task placed before us, with terminal illness, is the challenge of finding courage to face death's mystery ... of finding the inner strength that will support us in living while dying, rather than dying while we are yet alive.

For many people death is an emotional and spiritual crisis. *What is life all about? Was my life meaningful? Will I be remembered? How will I be remembered? Will my friend or loved one forgive me? Will I be totally dependent and a burden on others? Will I die in great pain? Will I die alone?* These are the palpable elements of emotional and spiritual suffering.

By examining the concerns and attitudes that you hold for your own death, you will be better prepared to help another to face theirs. This Unit provides you with the opportunity to ponder your own death and consider the issues and concerns that you may face at the end of your life. Will death come as an intruder or as a guest?

There are days we live
as if death were nowhere
in the background; from joy
to joy to joy, from wing to wing,
from blossom to blossom to
impossible blossom, to sweet impossible blossom.

Li-Young Lee (4)

EXERCISES

A. (45 minutes) *Relating to Death*

Write your responses to the following questions on the lines below. Then form small groups of three or four and share your responses. Finally, share with the large group.

- Has anyone close to you died?
- What did you learn from this experience?
- Did the individual change during the dying process?
- Did you change? If so, how?

What do you hope your death will be like? What do you imagine it will be like?

Do you believe there are any positive aspects of the dying process for the dying person or for their loved ones? If so, what are they?

What are your thoughts about what might come after death? What has influenced your thinking about this?

Have you ever discussed death with a dying person? What difficulties did/would you have in doing so?

B. (35 minutes) *Death as a Guest or Intruder*

Form groups of three or four in a circle. Leave an empty chair in the circle. Your trainer will lead this exercise.

Scenario 1: Death is sitting in the empty chair! Sit quietly without talking, and picture in your mind how death looks – its size, its color, how it feels, how it smells. Write your description on the lines below, and also write how you feel about death sitting there right now. You may also draw a picture of death to accompany your description. Share your experience with your small group and then with the large group.

My picture of death for Scenario 1:*

* This idea of drawing death came from Hospice of Summa Health System, Akron, Ohio.

Scenario 2: Death now stands outside the circle of chairs. You all agree to invite death into the group. Have one person in the group cordially invite death to sit in the empty chair as your welcomed guest. Repeat the directions above and share your experience with your small group. Did anything change for you? If so, what changed and why? Share some of your experience and feelings with the large group.

My new picture of death for Scenario 2:

my body
wasted by winter
if only I
like fields burned over
had hope for spring.

Lady Ise (5)

C. (60 minutes) *Receiving a Terminal Prognosis**

Your trainer will lead this exercise. Read each paragraph slowly and carefully, and then respond on the lines below. When you have completed the entire written exercise, share your thoughts with the large group.

It is Monday – a cold, dark, blustery, late winter afternoon. You have just arrived home after completing a series of medical tests designed to give you answers about why you have experienced pain in your side for several weeks. You will return to the doctor's office at the end of the week to hear the results. No one is home now, so you sit down to rest.

What are you thinking about?

____

____

____

____

What are you feeling?

____

____

____

Friday arrives and you have returned to your doctor's office. She tells you that you have a malignant tumor. They can't operate, but they can try chemotherapy and radiation treatments. After your appointment you sit in the waiting room for about 30 minutes. Finally, you leave the office and walk to your car. You sit there for a while still trying to absorb what your doctor has just told you.

What are you feeling?

____

____

____

____

* Adapted from Longaker C. Chapter 5. Understanding and responding to suffering. In: *Facing Death and Finding Hope: a guide to the emotional and spiritual care of the dying*. London: Random House; 1997; pp. 44–59.

What do you fear most?

When will you tell your family members? Who will you tell?

How will they react?

What friends will you tell? How will they react?

You think about how you have lived and what you expected to do for the next few years. How would you have lived life differently if you had known you might die in two to three years?

____

____

____

____

____

What activities will you continue? What activities will you stop? What do you want to finish?

____

____

____

____

____

____

____

____

____

____

It is now several months later. You have gone into the hospital a couple of days each month for treatments. You have had nausea and vomiting. You are still in pain and have other physical discomfort. Today, your doctor informed you that the treatments aren't working. There is nothing more they can try. There is no more chemotherapy, no more radiation. She has discussed hospice and palliative care with you.

What are you feeling?

____

____

What do you need to do?

What do you fear the most?

You are home now. You are so weak that you are unable to do many of the things you were used to doing. You spend much of your time lying down or in a wheelchair. Your family cares for your daily needs – bathing, dressing, feeding. Personnel from the hospice visit you regularly. You find them caring and compassionate.

What are you feeling?

What do you need?

What do you need to do?

When you look in the mirror you are dismayed to see how frail you look. Your body is wasted, and your skin is sallow and hangs loosely. Your hair is thin and straggly.

What are you feeling?

What do you need?

What do you need to do?

What do you fear the most?

____

____

____

____

____

You realize that there is not much time left now. Whom do you need to bid goodbye?

____

____

____

____

____

What do you want to say?

____

____

____

____

____

Who do you want in the room with you as you are dying?

____

____

____

____

____

What would you like them to do during your final hours?

____

____

What would you like them to do at the time of your death?

What will be in your heart and mind in the final moments of your life?

How did you feel doing this exercise? What did you learn about yourself?

(5 MINUTES) REFLECTIONS ON THIS UNIT

Journal Note for Unit 2.6

ASSIGNMENT

For the next session, complete the genogram found in Unit 3.1, Exercise A, and be prepared to share it with a partner.

ADDITIONAL RESOURCES

REFERENCES

1. Lief J. *Making Friends With Death: a Buddhist guide to encountering mortality*. Boston, MA: Shambhala; 2001.
2. Morris V. *Talking About Death Won't Kill You*. New York: Workman Publishing; 2001.
3. Singh KD. *Dying As a Spiritual Event. On Our Own Terms, Moyers on Dying*. Public Affairs Television, Inc., 2000. www.wnet.org/onourownterms/articles/spiritual2.html
4. Lee L-Y. In: *Blossoms*. www.ahapoetry.com/twanth1.html (accessed 23 July 2009).
5. Lady Ise. www.ahapoetry.com/twanth1.html (accessed 23 July 2009).

Part 3:
Understanding Ourselves in Service of the Dying Person

Humans are complex social beings who have bodies, personalities, lived pasts, spiritual lives, and networks of social, political, and cultural relationships. All of these dimensions influence and provide boundaries for our thoughts and actions. An important element in understanding a dying person is to understand clearly how these dimensions influence our behaviors and perceptions.

The Units in this Part provide an opportunity to explore and better understand how race, gender, age, personality, spirituality, and beliefs about the nature of suffering affect our own lives. This heightened understanding provides a framework for the compassionate care of others.

Unit 3.1: Social and Cultural Influences

KEY ISSUES

Ethnic and cultural differences, character, stereotyping, case study, code of ethics.

(10 minutes) Meditation

(10 minutes) Journal Note Share

> *Acknowledging the other in the moment, being with, and traveling along with the other is transcending differences.*
>
> Rozzano Locsin (1: 4)

INTRODUCTION

Every one of us, particularly during our formative years, has been strongly influenced by factors such as race, ethnicity, gender, family, socio-economic status, and education. These factors ultimately influenced the blueprint by which we approach life. Our behavior and life choices are also influenced by our temperament – for example, how we trust or mistrust others, how we are open and generous or closed and protective, whether or not we are self-directed, and how we give and receive information. Collectively, these distinctions are numerous and complex. They affect us in a myriad of ways, and make us the unique individuals we are. Not only do they provide us with a structure for the way we live our lives, but also they may shape our notions about the cause of illness and death, what constitutes appropriate end-of-life care, where and how our dying should take place, and what death means.

Although a dying individual may speak and appear much the same as you, it is erroneous to assume that there are no ethnic or cultural differences that could hinder effective care or the relationship. If you ascertain that the beliefs and values of the dying person differ significantly from yours, it is critical that you acknowledge and honor the other's ideas and do not attempt to persuade them to change. Behavior contrary to this is unethical for a caregiver. Rather than focusing on the differences, Locsin (1: 2) offers the following approach:

> Emphasizing cultural similarities rather than differences builds bridges toward understanding human beings as persons. The wisdom gained by knowing these similarities and differences honors and affirms the value of these persons as human beings.

Generalizations and cultural stereotyping must also be avoided. Although caregivers possess some knowledge about an individual's influential background, they must remember that not every individual in a population embraces all aspects of the belief system represented in the broader group. Use this knowledge as tentative and as a stimulus to learn about the particularity of the individual.

In this Unit you will have the opportunity to share and discuss your own ethnic and cultural background and your ideas about dying and death, you will contemplate the situation of Mei Lee, an elderly dying woman, and you will develop a code of ethics for caregivers.

EXERCISES

A. (40 minutes) *Construct a Genogram**

A genogram is a method of identifying your family tree and telling family stories. On the next page is a template of a genogram for you to complete (M = male, F = female). In the lines, place the first name of the individual. At the left you will find the request for other information, such as the ethnicity of the person (e.g. German), and the home town (e.g. Bigtown, Nevada or Lyons, France). On the children's lines, place the names according to the birth order in the family, and draw a circle around your own name. In the case of second or more marriages or significant relationships, give the year of divorce, death, or permanent separation, and the year of the next marriage or significant relationship.

When you have completed your genograms and story, share them with a partner, and then share your thoughts about this exercise with the large group.

* We wish to thank John Launer (2: 65–81) for first introducing us to the use of the genogram in narrative practice.

GENOGRAM

1) Grandparents: M ________ F ________ M ________ F ________

Ethnicity: ________ ________ ________ ________

Home: ________ ________ ________ ________

2) Parents: M ________ F ________

Home: ________ ________

Born ________ Died ________ Born ________ Died ________

3) Children in birth order (indicate M or F). Circle yourself

________ ________ ________ ________ ________ ________

4) You and spouse or significant other (indicate M or F)

____________ ____________

Born ________ Born ________

Home ________ Home ________

Divorce or end of relationship ____________

New marriage or relationship ____________ ____________

Born ________ Born ________

Home ________ Home ________

5) Children in birth order (indicate M or F)

________ ________ ________ ________ ________

Write a brief story about your genogram to illustrate how your ethnic, cultural, and immediate family background has influenced your development. Has your gender, education, or socio-economic situation played a role? How about your personal characteristics?

B. (45 minutes) *Case Study*

This is a large group activity. First, your trainer will ask for a volunteer to read the following case. Then discuss the case and the questions below.

> Mei Lee is an elderly woman of Chinese heritage. You meet her in the palliative care unit. She has a husband and two daughters. You learn that her family, particularly her husband, has assumed all decision making for her healthcare, and they insist that she should not be told that she is dying. They are making arrangements to have her discharged home, and are adamant that she should not die in the palliative care unit or in the hospice. When you visit her and speak to her she seldom looks at you directly, she always appears reserved and quiet, she never complains, and if she does speak it is mostly in Chinese.

What further information do you need?

____

____

____

____

____

How will you proceed?

____

____

____

____

____

C. (45 minutes) *Code of Ethics*

This is a large group activity. List on the chalkboard or chart paper those behaviors that you believe should be included in a *Caregivers' Code of Ethics* (e.g. "Never judge another's beliefs, values, rituals, or morals"). Copy your list onto the chart below. You will review this chart later to edit or expand it.

Caregivers' Code of Ethics

(5 MINUTES) REFLECTIONS ON THIS UNIT

Journal Note for Unit 3.1

ASSIGNMENT

(To be determined by trainer.)

ADDITIONAL RESOURCES

1. Callahan M, Kelley P. *Final Gifts: understanding the special needs and communication of the dying*. New York: Bantam Books; 1997.
2. Buchwald D, Caralis PV, Gany F *et al.* Caring for patients in a multicultural society. *Patient Care*. 1994; **28:** 105–23.
3. Waltman RE. Questions to ask senior patients. *Med Econ*. 2002; **25:** 29–30, 33.

REFERENCES

1. Locsin RC. Building bridges: affirming culture in health and nursing. *Holistic Nurs Pract*. 2000; **15:** 1–4.
2. Launer J. *Narrative-Based Primary Care*. Oxford: Radcliffe Medical Press; 2002.

Unit 3.2: Spiritual and Religious Influences

KEY ISSUES

Religious influences, secular beliefs, organized religion.

(10 minutes) Meditation

(10 minutes) Journal Note Share

> *... as people begin to share their spiritual thinking, what we will hear will be unique and powerful. Sometimes it will be joyful and empowering, at other times disturbing. Hopefully it will always be helpful.*
>
> Stephen Kliewer and John Saultz (1: 100)

INTRODUCTION

Since the earliest times, humankind has been strongly drawn toward religion and spirituality. As we noted earlier, the word "spirit" derives from the Latin *spiritus*, referring to the breath, moving air, or the life force. Also in that earlier Unit, you discovered how differently humans view spirituality and how they relate spirituality and religion. Furthermore, you learned that for many individuals, spirituality has to do with the meaning and purpose of life and with connections. It was further emphasized that in the quest for meaning most people seek something outside themselves, something greater than themselves, to guide them – a higher power or force, a superior being whom they respect and revere and obey or fear. Some find guidance in organized religion, while others find spiritual meaning in more secular or worldly entities such as nature, music, or commitment to family and community. These latter individuals are certainly not exempt from suffering intense spiritual needs and dilemmas.

When we look at the meaning of the word "*religion*" we see that it has a very different meaning to spirituality. It derives from the Latin *religio*, meaning a reverence for and union with the gods. In modern times we think of religion as an organized system of belief, worship, and rituals, such as the Muslim, Jewish, or Christian religions. And while most organized faith systems have at their core a belief in a divine or superhuman being or God, this is not true of all religions. Liz Flower, author of *The Elements of World Religions* (2: 1), provides us with the following brief and succinct account of these differences:

> Religions have either the one all-powerful God (Judaism, Christianity, Islam, Sikhism), or a pantheon of gods within which the One may be implicit (Hinduism, Shinto, primal religions) or indeed no God as such, but a state of transcendence with which one may escape from the sufferings of the world (Buddhism, Jainism) by following the teachings of the first propounder (and his successors) of that religion.

Keeping these distinctions in mind, caregivers must remember then that among human beings the image or meaning of God may differ dramatically. Some people believe in an all-seeing, all-powerful, loving God, while others see God as punishing and frightening. And for some a God does not exist at all. During the dying process, some individuals will lament that God has abandoned them or they have conflicted feelings about God's presence or existence, while others may experience a sudden spiritual epiphany. At times it becomes quite obvious that, as Hardwig (3: 28) notes, " … strong religious convictions are not [always] sufficient to ensure a good death or to endow the terminal phase of life with meaning, purpose, or validity."

Because religion often has a profound influence on a person's life and death, we have devoted this Unit to the examination of the many different religions. You will learn how the customs and rituals relating to dying and death vary from one faith tradition to another, and how people who are non-religious approach the dying process. Regardless of your own particular beliefs, becoming more well acquainted with the various religions will help you to understand better the person in your care.

It is not at all uncommon for a caregiver to see the need to explore the spiritual or religious beliefs of the dying person – not simply to satisfy their own curiosity, but also to ascertain how or why the individual's decisions or wishes are influenced by their beliefs. You may find that your belief systems are quite similar, or they may be at great odds. Regardless of the similarities or differences, the other's beliefs should never be challenged. In these latter instances or when you are not at all familiar with their religion, simply invite the dying person to "help you to understand" their beliefs. Exploring the other's beliefs is neither difficult nor intrusive if it is approached in a sensitive way, and we shall practice it in this Unit.

You may find that you cannot tolerate some of the other's beliefs. Rather than cause great discomfort for yourself or for a dying person, you may decide that it is best that you withdraw from caregiving and help to locate another caregiver. We must further emphasize that while you recognize certain practices as belonging to a particular faith, it is a mistake to believe that every individual who embraces that tradition or sect observes or practices exactly the same principles. When the influences of culture, ethnicity, and experience are integrated with any given faith, beliefs and values can be modified significantly. Again, this is a situation that can be explored.

EXERCISES

A. (60 minutes) *Panel Discussion*

Your trainer will invite individuals from the community who belong to different religious groups to form a panel that will present information about the beliefs, rituals and practices regarding dying and death in their particular faith system. Also on the panel will be one or more individuals who do not belong to an organized religion and who may or may not believe in a God. You should feel free to ask questions during the presentations. If a panel is not available, you can locate materials on the web or in libraries that describe the beliefs and rituals of the various faith systems with regard to dying and death. These can be used for discussion.

B. (30 minutes) *Reflecting on Your Own Spiritual Beliefs*

Form pairs or small groups and discuss the following questions. Share some of your thoughts with the large group.

- What are your spiritual roots?
- How have your spiritual beliefs changed over time?
- How have your spiritual beliefs shaped your relationship with yourself and others?
- What is your current spiritual practice?
- How has your spirituality/religion influenced your beliefs about dying and death?

C. (40 minutes) *Discussing Spirituality and Religion*

The following is an example of how you might begin to explore a dying person's spiritual/religious beliefs. With a partner, one person having the role of the caregiver and the other having the role of the dying person, practice the conversation as it is suggested below and then *switch roles*. You do not have to hold strictly to the example, but it is important to keep the questions open to encourage the other to continue the conversation. Then share your experience and ideas with the large group.

- You have been diagnosed with a terminal illness, and here you are now in [hospice/the palliative care unit]. I can well imagine what a worrying time this is for you.
- Tell me about other times in your life when you have faced very critical health situations. How and where did you find hope?
- What gives your life purpose and meaning?
- Do you consider yourself a spiritual person?
- Tell me about your spiritual beliefs.
- In the past, have you relied on your faith or religion to help you to cope with a life-threatening illness – either yours or that of a member of the family? Is your faith comforting for you now?
- Do you belong to an organized religion or community? How does that community support you?
- Are there religious or spiritual issues that are concerning you now?
- Do you have someone to talk to about your concerns? Would you like to talk to someone?
- Is there some way that I can help you with your concerns, or would you like me to contact someone for you to talk to?

(5 MINUTES) REFLECTION ON THIS UNIT

Journal Note for Unit 3.2

____

____

____

____

____

____

____

ASSIGNMENT

Write your responses to the following questions and then come to the next session prepared to discuss them.

1. What spiritual anguish did Ivan Ilyich suffer?
2. Was religion involved? If so, how? How did he feel about it?
3. What did he mean by the "black hole"?
4. How did he work through his losses?
5. What challenges you about any of the religions, their practices or beliefs?
6. Are there any religious beliefs that you cannot work with?
7. Are there any boundaries that you must draw?
8. How would you handle a situation where your own beliefs are in conflict with those of the dying person?
9. Where can you refer the dying person for spiritual/religious help?

ADDITIONAL RESOURCES

1. Kirkwood NA. *A Hospital Handbook on Multiculturalism and Religion*. Harrisburg, PA: Morehouse Publishing; 1993.
2. Thomason CL. Inclusive spirituality. *J Fam Pract.* 1999; **48:** 17–18.
3. Dunne T. Spiritual care at the end of life. *Hastings Center Report.* 2001; **31:** 22–6.
4. Muller W. *How, Then, Shall We Live? Four simple questions that reveal the beauty and meaning of our lives.* New York: Bantam Books; 1997.

REFERENCES

1. Kliewer D, Saultz J. *Healthcare and Spirituality*. Oxford: Radcliffe Publishing; 2006.
2. Flower l. *The Elements of World Religions*. Rockport, MA: Element Books; 1997.
3. Hardwig J. Spiritual issues at the end of life: a call for discussion. *Hastings Center Report.* 2000; **30:** 28–30.

Unit 3.3: The Nature of Loss and Suffering

KEY ISSUES

Losses and gains, suffering, grief, grief reaction.

(10 minutes) Meditation

(10 minutes) Journal Note Share

> *Although grief is not evenly apportioned, everyone lives with some. If we understand and accept grief as part of our humanity, our suffering will diminish.*
>
> Rodney Smith (1: 171)

INTRODUCTION

For human beings, loss is inevitable, and suffering is inevitable. At every turn in our lives, our personhood is vulnerable to assault and injury – our physical being, our family roles, our social and political roles, our relationships, our work, our faith, our past and future. Death – the loss of this life – is perhaps the greatest of losses, and suffering is its dire companion. Ira Byock (2: 82–3), author of *Dying Well*, speaks of this in the following passage:

> Personal stress or suffering of some extent is universal among people who are dying, even those who have no physical discomfort. It may range from subtle loss of interest in life and a pervasive sense of uneasiness to terrifying, agonizing torment. While easy passages from life do occur, for most people the months and weeks that precede the moment of their death involve effort and inner struggles as they confront the gradual loss of their abilities, roles, and relationships and as they work to achieve some equilibrium in the face of inexorable decline.

Clearly, dying was an agonizing torment for Ivan Ilyich. We were witness to all of his feelings and finally to his release. However, as Byock notes above, and as we related in Unit 2.6, not all people who are dying suffer as horribly as Ivan did. For those who have accepted that death and loss are inevitable, the journey can be quite tranquil. However, accepting death can be a very slow or very rapid process, in which not everyone succeeds (2).

Let us think about our own losses – some have been minor, some major. You may have lost your wallet or purse, experienced a divorce, or lost your job or your home. Perhaps a favorite pet, or a child, a relative, or a beloved friend died. Regardless of the significance of the loss, grief is the usual reaction and you probably remember it well. However, grief does not always come to us as intense sadness. It can appear in many different guises (e.g. anger, blame, guilt, jealousy, self-pity, fear, withdrawal, or depression). Over time, if grief is neglected, misunderstood, or unresolved, it closes down our hearts and becomes toxic to our entire being. Our suffering and painful emotions will continue until the threat to our personhood is removed or we accept it and deal with it.

On the brighter side of grief is the fact that, for many losses, there are ensuing gains. Most of us know someone who has experienced a divorce or the death of a spouse, leaving them not only alone, but perhaps nearly destitute. They were forced to take a new job in order to maintain their home and care for the family. However, this loss, as difficult as it was, may have moved them into a new and exciting career, one that they would never have dreamed of. In the medical world it is quite common to hear people who have survived a serious life-threatening disease or trauma say, "It was the best thing that ever happened to me." Through their near loss, they learned the meaning of life. Ivan Ilyich was forced to work through his losses himself, but he indeed found peace at the very end.

So that we may better understand the grief of the dying person in our care, it is important that we spend time understanding our own loss and grief reactions, and how we work through them, and that we discern any gains that may have resulted. This Unit gives you that opportunity and will also enable you to practice your skills in discussing these issues with others.

EXERCISES

A. (30 minutes) *Assignment from Unit 3.2*

This is a large group discussion of the questions in the assignment.

B. (60 minutes) *Personal Loss Graph**

The first line below is a timeline for your life. Write your birth date at the left end and the present year, date, and your age at the right end. The dot in the middle is the midpoint of your life so far. Along this line place short vertical lines or slashes for every loss you have suffered during your life. Number and label each event and your approximate age at that time. On the lines underneath the timeline, write the event number and then (a) the event, (b) the feelings or emotions it caused for you, (c) the length of time it took for you to work through your grief or if you still carry it with you, (d) what you gained from each loss, and (e) the result of the gain.

Timeline of My Life Losses

_______________________________ ■ _______________________________

Birth date Midpoint Current date/age

____

____

____

____

____

____

____

Review your timeline and life losses and gains with a partner, and then share some thoughts and feelings with the entire group.

C. (40 minutes) *Relationship with Loss*†

Your trainer will lead this exercise. At the end, you will have the opportunity to discuss the exercise with the entire group.

- Sit in a circle
- You will receive four pieces of colored paper (e.g. four yellow, four green, four blue, and four red slips), so 16 pieces in total. Place these on the table or on the floor in front of you.

---

* Adapted from: James JW, Friedman R. *The Grief Recovery Handbook*. New York: HarperCollins; 1998.

† This is an adaptation of an exercise which came from Frank Ostaseski and the Zen Hospice Project and was originally attributed to Rev. Dick Lentz, St. Vincent Hospice, Indianapolis, IN.

- Think about the material possessions that you love or appreciate in your life (e.g. jewelry, home, car, book, or other items). Select four that you most cherish, and write one of these on each piece of yellow paper. Sit silently and reflect on these four things and their importance to you.
- Think about the activities that you love or appreciate in your life (e.g. running, reading, kissing, swimming, or others). Select the four that are most important to you, and write one on each piece of green paper. Sit silently and reflect on these four activities.
- Think about the roles or identities that you have in your life (e.g. mother, engineer, bus driver, teacher, sister). Choose the four that are most important to you, and write one on each piece of blue paper. Sit silently and reflect on the importance of these roles in your life.
- Think about the relationships that you love and appreciate in your life (e.g. father, daughter, aunt, mother, or the names of individuals). Select the four that are most important to you, and write one on each piece of red paper. Sit silently and reflect on the love and appreciation that you feel for the four roles or individuals.
- Arrange all of the paper slips, in any order you choose, on the table or floor in front of you. Reflect on your selections and think about your relationship to each.
- As we all know, life losses can occur at any time and we have no control over them. The trainer will move around the circle and may take one or more of your pieces of paper and place them in the basket that he or she is carrying. Reflect on this loss.
- There are also times, such as during the loss of a job or money or a spouse, where we have some choice about the things we must give up. Select four pieces of paper of any color and place them in the trainer's basket. Look at the remaining slips and reflect on your relationship with what has been lost and what remains.
- Imagine now that you are facing a life-threatening illness. You know that loss is inevitable. Your neighbor, acting as that threat, will pick one yellow slip of paper, one green slip, one blue slip, and one red slip and place them in the basket that the trainer is holding. Now look at the remaining slips and reflect on your relationship with what has been lost and what remains.
- Now death arrives. All of your remaining papers go into the trainer's basket – or perhaps death passes you by. Look at the empty space and reflect on your relationship with what has been lost.

In the large group, discuss the following questions:

a) What issues, fears, and concerns arose for you with each loss?
b) How did you think/feel/respond when the trainer took one slip of paper from you? Did they take the "right "one? Is there a "right" one?
c) What were the easiest items to lose? What were the most difficult to lose?
d) How did you feel when your neighbor, representing a life-threatening illness, took your papers?
e) What did you think/feel when death took all of your remaining papers? If death passed you by, how did you feel?
f) When did this experience stop being a game?

The Ship*

I am standing upon a sea shore. A ship at my side spreads her white sails to the morning breeze and starts for the blue ocean. She is an object of beauty and strength and I watch her until at length she hangs like a speck of white cloud just where the sea and sky come down to mingle with each other. Then someone at my side says, "There she's gone." Gone where? Gone from my sight – that is all.

She is just as large in mast and hull and spar as she was when she left my side, and just as able to bear her load of living freight to a place of destination. Her diminished size is in me, not her; and just at the moment when someone at my side says, "There, she's gone", there are other eyes watching her coming, and other voices ready to take up the glad shout "Here she comes!"

And this is dying.

Henry Van Dyke

* After considerable research by many writers, there seems to be consensus that Henry Van Dyke is the author of *The Ship*. However, the original work or date is not cited.

(5 MINUTES) REFLECTIONS ON THIS UNIT

Journal Note for Unit 3.3

____

____

____

____

____

ASSIGNMENT

(To be determined by trainer.)

ADDITIONAL RESOURCES

1. Doka KJ, Davidson JD, eds. *Living with Grief: who we are, how we grieve*. Philadelphia, PA: Brunner/Mazel, for Hospice Foundation of America; 1998.
2. Caplan S, Lang G. *Grief's Courageous Journey: a handbook*. Oakland, CA: New Harbinger Publications; 1985.
3. Westberg G. *Good Grief: a constructive approach to the problem of loss*. Minneapolis, MN: Fortress Press; 1971.
4. Viorst J. *Necessary Losses*. New York: Fireside; 1998.

REFERENCES

1. Smith R. *Lessons From the Dying*. Somerville, MA: Wisdom Publications; 1998.
2. Byock I. *The Four Things That Matter Most*. New York: Free Press; 2004.

Part 4:
Ways of Helping the Dying Person

Accompanying the dying person on their journey can be enhanced through the awareness and sensitive application of a wide variety of approaches that can provide comfort and emotional support to the dying person.

The Units in this Part provide practice in these approaches. They range from communication skills such as mindful listening, compassionate presence, and responsive processes of relating, through the power of witnessing to the importance of rituals, prayers, and art forms for the relief of suffering.

Unit 4.1: Fundamentals of Communication

KEY ISSUES

Body language, congruence of communication, effective questions.

(10 minutes) Meditation

(10 minutes) Journal Note Share

> *The slogan "Pay attention to details" is about looking into the details of our behavior and seeing how they reflect underlying attitudes that we may not be aware of, how they reinforce such attitudes, and what they communicate to others.*
>
> Judith Lief (1: 136)

INTRODUCTION

At the very first visit, the caregiver's primary goal is to begin to develop a comfortable and trusting relationship with the dying person. This requires maintaining an open mind, heart, and spirit, and expressing deep interest and understanding. Cultivating these dispositions relies almost exclusively on communicating effectively. Many individuals seem to make close personal connections easily and naturally, but for those who find it challenging, we firmly believe that these skills can be learned. The key elements are authenticity and compassion, along with the willingness to learn and practice.

Central to the caring relationship is not only "paying attention to the details of our behavior" and knowing what to say and when to say it, but also being mindful about what the other is saying and not saying. Let us begin by thinking about the physical behaviors that are a big part of communication – nonverbal or body language. It is said that all communication between human beings starts in the eyes and the rest of the body, and that body language constitutes 50% or more of what we communicate. In view of this information, it is critical that caregivers understand what messages their bodies are sending to the ill person, and what nonverbal messages the ill person is displaying.

> *Hidden from all*
> *I will speak to you*
> *without words.*
> *No one but you*
> *will hear my story*
> *even if I tell it in the middle*
> *of a crowd.*
>
> Rumi (2: 112)

We signal our attitudes and our feelings through movements of our eyes, head, arms, fingers and legs as well as our facial muscles, our crossed limbs, and our shoulders and other body parts. When speaking of basic attending skills, we are talking about those behaviors, particularly with our eyes and upper body, which let the other know that we are with them and ready to hear them. Depending on your physical and emotional states, body language occurs in clusters of signals and postures that can emphasize, create confliction, or negate your verbal message. Whether or not your nonverbal message matches your verbal message is also telling behavior. Other nonverbal elements that can significantly affect the relationship include the following:

- positioning of the body relative to the other
- the size and shape of the body
- skin color and texture
- cleanliness
- loudness, pitch, and texture of the voice
- speed of speaking
- sweating, oral and body odors and other scents.

In Unit 4.2 we shall focus on what to say and how to say it, but here in this Unit, in addition to body language, we shall also turn our attention to how we use questions and statements. Just think how often you ask questions and how differently you construct them. Clearly, questions serve several purposes – to gain attention, to share information, to obtain information, or to start the other person thinking or visualizing. In our work with dying people we use questions for all these purposes, and it is exceedingly important that you know how to use questions that will help the dying person to open their mind and heart to healing. Too often, however, questions – particularly *why* questions – can put the other person on the defensive. *How*, *when*, or *where* questions are generally not so provocative. Sometimes it is not so much the question we ask as the way in which we ask it. So we should be careful about how we pose questions, and it is even more useful to know how to change questions into statements that are not in any way threatening. Using statements rather than questions can be far more valuable for obtaining information and stimulating the other to elaborate on a topic. For example, instead of asking, "Why are you so quiet?", we can make the statement "You are quiet today." A statement such as this tends to encourage the other to share his mood. Another way to encourage elaboration is to begin with phrases such as "Tell me about ...", "It seems that you ...", "Would you share with me ...", or "I would be really interested in hearing more about ...". You will practice other kinds of statements and questions in the next Unit.

EXERCISES

A. (30 minutes) *Nonverbal Language**

This is a large group activity. The participants should sit in a circle. The trainer will ask for volunteers to demonstrate the following elements of nonverbal language.

1. Use basic attending skills – simple behaviors of the head, face, and eyes only – to say:
   - I am listening and I want you to continue
   - I am with you, I am present to you
   - I don't agree with you
   - You're thinking all wrong
   - You are disgusting.
2. Add the shoulders, torso, and arms to say:
   - I am bored
   - I am present to you
   - I am relaxed and comfortable with you
   - I would rather be somewhere else right now
   - I really don't want to talk about it
   - I'm uncomfortable with you.
3. Use the whole body to say:
   - I'm ready to hear whatever you want to tell me
   - I really need to leave – I have another appointment
   - You're too close to me
   - I'm bored and I want to leave
   - I'm uncomfortable with what you're talking about.

* It is important to note that the meaning of body language may not be the same in all cultures.

B. (15 minutes) *Congruence of Verbal and Nonverbal Language*

In communication, congruence means that the body language matches or affirms the spoken message. Incongruence means that the body language is counter to the spoken message, even to the point of negating it. If there is disagreement between our body language and our spoken language, the body will almost always reveal the truth. Congruence only occurs when the individual is being real and genuine. Remain in the large group circle. With the following spoken lines, volunteers should demonstrate first congruence and then incongruence:

- I am glad to be able to visit you today
- I am feeling better today
- I am glad you came to visit today.

Share with the group other examples of congruent and incongruent communication.

- If you observe in the storyteller incongruence between their spoken message and their verbal message, how can you address it? Why is it important to address it?

C. (25 minutes) *Kinds and Purposes of Questions*

Remain in the same large group circle. Remember that the purposes of questions are to gain attention, to share information, to obtain information, or to start the other person thinking or visualizing. On the lines below write what you believe is the purpose of each of the following questions and statements:

- How was it for you growing up?

____

- Tell me about your work.

____

- If you could choose your work again, would you choose differently?

____

- Would you share some of your favorite childhood memories with me?

____

- Was your life different from what you thought it would be?

____

- What do you consider to be your greatest achievement in life?

____

- Tell me about a painful loss in your life. How did you deal with it? What was a good thing that came from that loss?

Now it's your turn. On the lines below, write a question that you believe would represent each of the stated purposes. Share these with the group.

Gain attention:

____

____

____

Obtain information:

____

____

____

Share information:

____

____

____

Start the other person thinking or visualizing:

____

____

____

Were some of your questions open-ended and were some closed so that they could be answered with a simple "yes" or "no"? What does this mean? When would you use each type of question?

D. (40 minutes) *Practice Using Questions*

The trainer or a participant should volunteer to tell a story about a difficult time or incident in their life. This storyteller should share only one or two sentences at a time and then pause, giving each group member the opportunity to ask a question. The storyteller should give very short "yes" or "no" or one-word responses to closed questions and not elaborate, so that everyone really understands the effect of closed questions. Determine the type of question that was asked and whether it was the appropriate kind of question to ask at that time. If not, correct it.

E. (20 minutes) *Practice Using Statements*

Change each question below to a statement, and then share your statements in the large group.

Why are you crying?

____

____

Where did you work?

____

____

What do you want to happen for you next?

____

____

(5 MINUTES) REFLECTIONS ON THIS UNIT

Journal Note for Unit 4.1

____

____

____

____

____

ASSIGNMENT

(To be determined by the trainer.)

REFERENCES

1. Lief JL. *Making Friends With Death: a Buddhist guide to encountering mortality*. Boston, MA: Shambhala; 2001.
2. Kolm AM, Mafi M, translators. *Rumi: hidden music*. London: Thorsons/HarperCollins Publishers; 2001.

Unit 4.2: Compassionate Presence, Mindful Listening, and Effective Responding

KEY ISSUES

Presence, listening mindfully, paraphrasing, empathy, sympathy.

(10 minutes) Meditation

(10 minutes) Journal Note Share

> *The friend who can be silent with us in a moment of despair or confusion, who can stay with us in our hour of grief and bereavement, who can tolerate not knowing, not curing, not healing, and face with us the reality of our powerlessness, – that is a friend who cares.*
>
> Henri J.M. Nouwen (1: 34)

INTRODUCTION

Effective caregiving is absolutely grounded in the act of *being with* the dying person – being *present*. "Well", you might respond, "if I go to visit that individual I am present. I'm there, aren't I?" But it is not so simple. Too often we take our everyday "busy-ness" with us – our own concerns, our need to talk, judge, and influence, our need to be in control. What the dying person needs is our undivided whole self who has put aside personal life matters, needs, and wounds in order to be *present* to their woundedness – their physical condition, their emotional turmoil, and their spiritual fears and concerns. When we visit, we must be ready to offer our open and peaceful heart and mind and spirit. The critical skill underlying *presence* is mindful listening. We talked about this in Unit 2.2. Again you might respond "Of course I listen." However, mindful listening and really hearing what the other is saying is another issue that is not as simple as it may sound. Hugh Prather (2: 108), in his book *I Touch the Earth and The Earth Touches Me*, speaks succinctly of mindful listening:

> I can listen to someone without hearing him. Listening is fixing my attention only on the other person. Hearing requires that I listen inside me as I listen to him. Hearing is a rhythm whereby I shuttle between his words and my experience. It includes hearing his entire posture: his eyes, his lips, the tilt of his head, the movement of his fingers. It includes hearing his tone of voice and his silences. And hearing also includes attending to my reactions, such as the "sinking feeling" I get when the other person has stopped hearing me.

When we share a problem or concern with another individual, we don't always want answers or solutions – what we want from the *other* is simply to hear us, because generally, as we hear ourselves in the presence of the *other's* silence, we will arrive at our own answers. We all recognize the sinking feeling Prather speaks of when we realize that the *other* has turned off and is not really present to us. The ability to listen actively, generously, and mindfully without interfering or judging is challenging to our human nature, but critical to our relationships. Too often, as we listen to the other, we sit there rehearsing how we will respond, or we try to *psychologize* (i.e. we try to figure out what we believe that person is *really* thinking or feeling). Perhaps we are working on how to tell them they are wrong-thinking and we are planning how to advise them or influence them to change their thinking, or maybe we change the subject completely. **All of these tendencies are blocks to active mindful listening**. As we noted in a previous unit, meditation is a practice that helps us to still or quiet the mind and focus attention so that we can be present. Active mindful listening does not mean merely sitting silently without opening our mouth, or not thinking. Rather, it requires us to hear accurately what the other is communicating and then collaborate with them in ways that clarify meaning, acknowledge feelings, and aid them in constructing a complete and meaningful story.

There is a thread from the heart to the lips
where the secret of life is woven.
Words tear the thread.
but in silence
the secrets
speak.

Rumi (3: 96)

In Unit 4.1 we worked on fundamental communication skills – the messages that our bodies send, synchronizing verbal and nonverbal languages, basic attending skills such as eye contact, body position and movements that encourage the storyteller, and the effective use of questions. In this Unit we shall work on more advanced communication skills that will enable you to establish caring relationships not only with a dying patient, but also with everyone in your life. The following are three basic kinds of responses that keep the storytelling open and moving forward. They all depend on your ability to listen mindfully.

Paraphrasing

This is used to keep the story going, to clarify information, and to check for accuracy. It does not involve parroting the other's words, but instead rephrasing them as in the following example:

Storyteller: My brother called. He wants to see me. He hasn't spoken to me in 20 years! (silence)

Caregiver: After such a long time, your brother wants to visit.

(Here the storyteller knows that you have heard him or her accurately.)

Responding to content, meaning, and feeling

Storyteller: My brother called. He wants to see me. He hasn't spoken to me in 20 years! Why now? What does he want? (silence)

Caregiver: Your brother's call (content) was a real surprise to you (feeling) and it perplexes you (meaning).

(You have kept the communication open, and even if you are not quite accurate with your response, the teller will probably just correct you and continue with the story.)

Responding with sympathy or empathy

Often the words "sympathy" and "empathy" are confused or used interchangeably. The terms do not have the same meaning, and in order to learn how to respond with empathy a caregiver must recognize the differences. Sympathy tends to *block* communication when the responder immerses him- or herself in the sorrow or concern expressed by the teller. In this case, the response comes from a place outside of or away from and perhaps superior to the other person's situation. Most often, the responder "takes ownership" of the feeling that the teller has expressed. Empathy, on the other hand, is both a cognitive and affective skill which expresses a feeling of "walking beside" the other person in their anger, pain, joy, or grief, rather than in it. Expressing empathy requires one to perceive the source, depth, and breadth of the other's experience, and to communicate that understanding, providing a "mirror" that reflects all that one observes and hears in the other's story. The key is to take off one's own lenses and see through the other's eyes. Getting it right requires practice.

Storyteller: I can't die yet. What will my family do? There will be no one to take care of them. (silence)

1. Caregiver: (sympathetic response) "I'm sorry."
   (This is a superior or external position which can suggest "I'm glad it's not me.")
2. Caregiver: (assuming ownership) "Oh my, I don't want to die (with tears in the eyes). I'm so scared of dying."
   (Sympathetic responses steal away emotions from the teller and block further storytelling.)
3. Caregiver: (empathic response) "Leaving your family while you are so young is very worrisome for you."
   (Empathic responses honor the teller's meaning and feelings, and leave space for continued storytelling.)

EXERCISES

A. (30 minutes) *Practice Responding*

This is a whole group activity. First, each person should write a response as indicated to each statement. Then form a circle consisting of the whole group, and share your responses. The goal in each section is to keep the dialogue open so that the dying person will continue to talk.

1. Write a paraphrase for each of the following statements:

   - The pains in my head are so bad today, I just want to stay in my room in the dark and not talk.

     ____

     ____

     ____

   - I don't want to stay here in the hospital, I just want to go home.

     ____

     ____

     ____

     ____

- The doctor said that my test results look a little better this week.

2. Respond to content, meaning, and feeling.

   - All of these people coming in and out of my room at all times of the day and night drives me crazy!

   - I'm so happy – my son will arrive here on Tuesday!

   - I dread having my children see me like this. My little ones may not even know me without my hair.

3. Respond with sympathy and empathy. Describe what happens to the dialogue with each kind of response.

   - During your visit to a young terminally ill father, he sobs, "I don't want to die. I want to see my little boy grow up."

Sympathy:

____

____

____

____

Empathy:

____

____

____

____

- You meet your neighbor in the grocery store and you realize that he is very happy about something. He tells you that his doctor has just told him that his cancer is in remission.

Empathy:

____

____

____

____

Sympathy:

____

____

____

____

B. (25 minutes) *Advanced Skills*

Form dyads and practice the kind of responses that you have just learned. Each person gives a statement and the partner responds. Take turns and repeat several times. Discuss each response with regard to its accuracy, its effectiveness, how it felt, if it kept the communication open, and how to correct it.

C. (75 minutes) *Witnessing Another's Story**

You may change partners or retain the same partner. Decide which partner will be the first storyteller.

(5 minutes) Each person will have 5 minutes to tell a brief story about a serious illness or another traumatic event in their life. As the storyteller, during your story give the listener opportunities to respond or ask questions. As the listener, use all the new communication skills that you have learned. Pay attention to your body language and how you use questions, and always try to respond with empathy.

(5 minutes) When the first storyteller has finished, write as follows:

- The storyteller writes how it felt to tell the story and how the listener responded, and how comfortable the storyteller felt and why.
- The listener writes how it felt to hear the story and then respond to the storyteller, and how comfortable or uncomfortable they felt.

Storyteller:

Listener:

* We want to acknowledge that we first encountered this particular form of witnessing exercise while attending a workshop on narrative medicine conducted by Dr. Rita Charon and her colleagues at Columbia University, College of Physicians and Surgeons.

Do <u>not</u> share your writing at this time.

(10 minutes) Switch roles and repeat the exercise.
Storyteller:

Listener:

(10 minutes) When both stories and the writing are completed, each person writes about the other's story as follows. *Using your partner's voice*, write a short essay, poem, or journal entry, or a letter to someone in the story.

(15 minutes) Share your writings with your partner. **Note:** Do not hesitate to inform your partner about any uncomfortable moments in the interview and what caused them. Be sensitive, genuine, and courageous. This is an important learning activity in your preparation as a caregiver.

(40 minutes) Convene the large group. Each pair then shares their writings in the following way:

- The first listener shares how it felt to hear the story.
- The storyteller shares how it felt to tell their story, and comments on the listener's skills.
- The listener then asks the partner's permission to share the listener's composition about their story. Everyone is encouraged to agree to this, but a refusal must be honored.
  The storyteller should comment on the accuracy of the composition and how it felt to hear it.
- Repeat with the other partner.

Discuss this exercise in its entirety in the large group.

On the following lines, write what you need to learn and how you will practice your skills.

____

____

____

____

____

____

____

Caregiver's Prayer

Help me to remember that there is little I need to say and a lot I need to hear.
Help me to remember that I have little to teach and a lot to learn.
Help me to remember that sometimes the most important thing I can give is simply my presence, and sometimes nothing more is even wanted.
Help me to remember that all my education, all my training, and all my experience must always be secondary to my presence.
Help me to remember that I must accept and reaccept and reaccept and reaccept the uniqueness of the individual before me.
Help me to remember that I am not here for me; I am here for another.

Douglas C. Smith (4: 172)

(5 MINUTES) REFLECTIONS ON THIS UNIT

Journal Note for Unit 4.2

____

____

____

____

ASSIGNMENT

Complete Exercises A and B in Unit 4.3, and be prepared to discuss them in the next session.

ADDITIONAL RESOURCES

1. Wheatley MJ. Good listening. *Ions Noetic Sciences Rev*. 2002; **July-August:** 14–17.

REFERENCES

1. Nowen JM. *The Wounded Healer*. New York: Image Books; 1972.
2. Prather H. *I Touch the Earth, the Earth Touches Me*. New York: Doubleday & Co; 1972.
3. Kolm AM, Mofi M, translators. *Rumi: hidden music*. London: Thorsons/HarperCollins Publisher; 2001.
4. Smith DC, Chapin TJ. *Spiritual Healing*. Madison, WI: Psycho-Spiritual Publications; 2000.

Unit 4.3: Fears and Assumptions About Death

KEY ISSUES

Personal assumptions about death.

(10 minutes) Meditation

(10 minutes) Journal Note Share

> *The minister who has come to terms with his own loneliness and is at home in his own house is a host who offers hospitality to his guests. He gives them a friendly space where they may feel free to come and go, to be close and distant, to rest and to pray, to talk and be silent, to eat and to fast. The paradox indeed is that hospitality asks for the creation of an empty space where the guest can find his own soul.*
>
> Henri J.M. Nouwen (1: 92)

INTRODUCTION

You and I do not know about death; it is yet a mystery to us. But there is much we need to learn about the journey of the dying – how those who are dying deal with the reality of their approaching death, what they fear and need, what are the hindrances to their healing, and where hope lies for them. From the moment of our birth we have learned to fear death – from our parents, from our religion or other cultural beliefs, from our own near-death experiences, or from the death of a loved one. According to Ronald Smith (2: 65), "Fears collect in those areas of our lives where we are ignorant and have little clarity. And when our time to die comes upon us, all the fears we have accumulated come with it." Smith suggests that rather than remaining stalled on the same old fearful pathway, we can use our fears as signals that we need to heal those tortured places in our minds and hearts. In this

Unit we shall again face those buried fears of death head on, and practice ways to move them into a more peaceful place.

The renowned palliative care physician, Ira Byock (3: 4), proposes that although the dying person may indeed face a great many fears, their uppermost concern involves the people they love, and that "the specter of death reveals our relationships to be our most precious possessions." Through his many years caring for the dying, Byock states that he has learned that four simple statements "enliven all important relationships." In your work as a caregiver perhaps you will have the opportunity to encourage the dying person to express these four important statements to their loved ones:

> Please forgive me.
> I forgive you.
> Thank you.
> I love you.

For all of us, the only certain feature of the journey into death is uncertainty. Some deaths, of course, are immediate and often tragic, the result of instantaneous cardiac failure or perhaps a trauma of another sort, and in these instances we are denied the time to declare our love or say our goodbyes. For those individuals who are plagued with a disease such as multiple sclerosis or perhaps some form of cancer, where remission is short-term and only partial, death seems to linger forever in the shadows. For others, the prognosis of death may be imminent, within weeks or months. Regardless of the length of time or circumstance, for many people the journey is not an easy one. We each suffer our own fears and needs, and when our time of dying arrives, we come face to face with the assumptions that we have made about death. Judith Lief (4: 31–40), in her book *Making Friends with Death*, organizes these assumptions into five basic patterns which we have summarized as follows:

> *The Great Oblivion/The Great Rest*
> This assumption is that death is a state of utter oblivion, blackness, or lack of consciousness. If we hold this pattern we avoid death through blinders and routines, keeping the reality of death at arm's length. For some this state of lost consciousness is terrifying, while for others this view is hopeful, as it is a release from pain and struggle. For yet others, oblivion is a hopeful view. It is the time to lay down all of life's pain and struggle and find absolute rest.
>
> *The Great Insult/The Great Answer*
> In this pattern we view death as an insult, a mistake, a punishment. We are angry that death has to happen – it's not right. Here death is totally

unknown territory and impenetrable. We cannot figure it out and we are afraid of it. So we try to outsmart death with the right potions and pills, look for the genetic death code, eliminate all disease and live forever. We fight death at every step. In the very end we hope that the pieces of the puzzle will all fall into place and we will finally unravel the great mystery of life.

The Great Loss/The Great Reward
In this pattern we see death as a threat to every single thing we have gathered together throughout our entire life – our earthly possessions, our emotions, our intellectual and spiritual possessions, our insights, our accomplishments, our experiences or drama, our memories, and our bodies. We ward off death by accumulating more and more. Our hope is that although we may lose all that we have in this life, we will receive far greater rewards after we die, which serve as a sign of our worthiness. Or if we have been unsuccessful in life, our hope is to be rewarded in the afterlife, as we rightfully deserve.

The Great Departure/The Great Reunion
Here death separates us from our loved ones, our friends, our enemies, our casual acquaintances, our parents, our children, our pets, everyone. We cannot turn back or ever again see the faces of those we have left behind. Thus we cling to our relationships, we hang on for dear life, or perhaps we avoid forming relationships altogether. Our hope may be for reunion after death or perhaps union with a mystical being or force, or principle such as love and peace.

The Great Interruption/The Great Completion
Here death is the threat of unfinished business and we are not in control. We cannot count on completing what we have started. If getting things done is how we define ourselves, then not being able to do so is torture. We can no longer keep death at bay by keeping occupied. Our hope is that somehow death will bring true completion, and that life will come full circle.

The Butterfly

There is a story about a man who saw a butterfly trying unsuccessfully to free itself from its cocoon. Feeling very sorry to see the butterfly struggle, the man cut the cocoon free. But the butterfly couldn't fly,

> *and in fact died very quickly. The man later learned that cutting away the cocoon was the worst thing he could have done. He found out, only too late, that a butterfly needs to struggle to free itself from its cocoon in order to develop the muscles to fly. By robbing him of the struggle, the man made him too weak to live.*
>
> Author Unknown

As a caregiver you may meet individuals who demonstrate some of the patterns Lief describes above, and we hope that our summaries give you some notion as to what that individual is thinking and how they may eventually resolve their concerns. However, you must strive to remember the message of the butterfly. As we have emphasized many times, any attempts to influence the dying person's thinking or believe that it is your mission to be the fixer or savior will only potentially cause serious distress. We are not healers or saviors. Likewise, physicians and other healthcare professionals are not healers or saviors. Fortunately, these learned professional caregivers can provide palliative medicines and offer hope for a pain-free journey, but as for the emotional and spiritual aspects of dying, the best that any of us can do is to create a safe and empty space where the dying person can find his own soul and "free himself from his own cocoon." In Units 4.1 and 4.2 we laid the groundwork for effective communication. This Unit provides you with the opportunity to practice your skills, and challenges you to explore your own assumptions and fears about death.

EXERCISES

A. (30 minutes) *Fears about Death*

This was assigned at the end of the previous Unit. On the lines below, write down the fears you believe most people have about dying and death. Place an **X** next to those you possess, and note how and when they developed. Share your responses with a partner, and then discuss them in the large group.

____

____

____

____

____

____

What might make the idea of dying more bearable for you?

B. (30 minutes) *Assumptions about Death*

This exercise was assigned in the previous Unit. Which of Lief's patterns most closely fit(s) your view of death? Do you have other assumptions about death? How did you come to think in this way? Write your responses on the following lines. Share your thoughts in the large group.

C. (45 minutes) *Three Case Studies*

Imagine that you are paying a visit to each of the individuals in the following cases. Read each case introduction and describe how you would proceed and why. In the large group, discuss each case in turn.

1. Anne is a 38-year-old woman with a loving husband and two small children. She has end-stage pancreatic cancer, and she is deteriorating quite rapidly. Today you note that she seems much more depressed than she was last week, and quite reluctant to talk.

   ____

   ____

   ____

   ____

   ____

   ____

   ____

   ____

   ____

   ____

2. Roger is a 56-year-old man with a wife and a teenage son. He was diagnosed several years ago with Lou Gehrig's disease (ALS). His disease has now progressed to the point where he is confined to his bed. He has increased difficulty breathing and speaking due to the beginning of respiration paralysis. He waves you to his bedside and whispers in snatches "Isn't this a wonderful day?"

   ____

   ____

   ____

   ____

   ____

   ____

3. Henry is a 76-year-old man who only 2 months ago was diagnosed with very rapidly growing lung cancer. His wife is aging, and he has four grown and loving children and many grandchildren who all live in the area and visit him regularly. No one in the family shares their innermost thoughts or feelings. No one, including Henry's doctor, has told him in so many words that death is near. He is now very weak and confined to his bed. He has come to welcome your visits, and today as you sit down next to him, he suddenly takes hold of your arm and pulls you toward him and whispers to you "I'm not going to make it, am I?"

D. (25 minutes) *A Meditation Into Death and Love*

Your trainer will lead this meditation. Let's begin with a peaceful sitting meditation that you now know very well. Focus on your breath. Feel the air move in and out. Feel your abdomen rising and falling. You are centered and totally quiet. Feel your body softening and releasing. Feel peace entering your being. Rest here in your center for a while. Enjoy this quiet peaceful place, just watching the breath move in and out, feeling the peace.

Feel your body softening more. Honor your body. Thank your body for holding you, for protecting you. Slowly, slowly let go of your body, move out of it. You don't need it here. Let it go. Slowly let it go. There is no solid structure, only a feeling of softness and openness. You are floating free. You are safe and content. No body, no constraints, only slow soft fluid motion in empty space. Let go into this warm safe comforting peaceful place. You feel the love here.

The light here is soft and peaceful. Let go into the soft light, into the empty space. Dissolve into the light and the empty space. Be one with the soft color of love. Let go of any thoughts of life, images of life. There is no life. Just rest here in the soft peaceful light. It is peaceful and restful here, loving. You are safe here, floating and letting go. You are floating in the warm, loving, peaceful light.

Awareness dissolves into light and endless space.
You can feel yourself now connecting with the whole universe – floating with the whole universe, floating in the loving light – each breath melting into the light, into the universe.

You are floating free in the light and love.
You are part of the universe, part of the soft and peaceful light, part of the love.
You are light. You are love.

(5 MINUTES) REFLECTIONS ON THIS UNIT

Journal Note for Unit 4.3

____

____

____

____

____

ASSIGNMENT

Interview two or three friends or family members about how they view death. Ask them to first read Lief's five patterns as they are summarized in this Unit. Discuss which one(s) best fit their viewpoint and why. Tell them that this is part of your training and you will need to take notes about your discussion. Assure them that their name and other personal information will remain completely confidential. Come to the next session prepared to discuss your findings with the large group.

ADDITIONAL RESOURCES

1. Fife RB. Are existential questions for terminally ill patients? *J Palliat Med.* 2002; **5:** 815–17.

REFERENCES

1. Nouwen HJM. *The Wounded Healer*. New York: Image Books; 1972.
2. Smith R. *Lessons From the Dying*. Somerville, MA: Wisdom Publications; 1998.
3. Byock I. *The Four Things That Matter Most*. New York: Free Press; 2004.
4. Lief J. *Making Friends with Death: a Buddhist's guide to encountering mortality*. Boston, MA: Shambhala; 2001.

Unit 4.4: Narratives of Suffering

KEY ISSUES

Suffering, stories, spiritual questions.

(10 minutes) Meditation

(10 minutes) Journal Note Share

> *Healing, in the narrative sense, does not come through the "laying on of hands" ... rather, healing is in the "laying on of ears."*
>
> Romanoff and Thompson (1: 31)

INTRODUCTION

Suffering is no stranger to us; it has been a lifelong companion. We know its pain, its yearning, its grief. It has not been limited to physical pain – consider the jobs lost, the child's fearful illness, the work failed or unfinished, the wounded hearts we have endured. Eric Cassell (2: 643) speaks of the many dimensions of suffering as follows:

> Suffering is ultimately a personal matter. ... Patients sometimes report suffering when one does not expect it, or do not report suffering when one does expect it. ... All the aspects of personhood – the lived past, the family's lived past, culture and society, roles, the instrumental dimension, association and relationships, the body, the unconscious mind, the political being, the secret life, the perceived future, and the transcendent dimension – are susceptible to damage and loss.

Most certainly the prognosis of death is the supreme injury, and it has the potential to engender much or all that Cassell describes. It can threaten the very nature of who we are and what gives our lives meaning and purpose, and it can rob us of hope. The Buddhists would remind us that suffering is an indication that we have attached ourselves to things that are destined to cease. But in the last days of life how do we let go? How do we mend the wounded soul? How do we find hope in the midst of such loss? Stephen Levine, best known for his work on death and dying (3: 3) in his book *Healing into Life and Death*, describes what he has learned through his many years of caring for the dying:

> For years our work with the dying has mostly been an encouragement to open fully to this moment in which all life is expressed, that the optimum preparation for death is a whole-hearted opening to life even in its subtlest turnings and changes. But it turned out for some that this opening to life did not pave the way to death but instead resulted in a deepening access to levels of healing beyond imagination.

Once again, recognizing that we are not fixers or saviors, how do we, as caregivers, help those who are dying to open fully to this moment? As we have emphasized repeatedly in this training, our answer is that we listen mindfully to the dying person's stories. Romanoff and Thompson (1: 311) summarize for us all that we have worked on:

> The attitude of the listener toward the narrative substantially influences how the story is told and may inhibit or facilitate the narrative process. Narrative responses can be suppressed if the listener attempts to control the interaction by pursuing a particular line of inquiry, or if specific questions are used that reflect the listener's interests rather than the narrator's priorities. Narrative disinterest is also communicated when the listener interrupts or redirects the story, hurries responses, or attempts to elicit "facts" rather than the storied accounts that may or may not represent the objective truth. When the attitude of the listener is receptive, the narrator is given freedom to pursue topics of his or her choice, introduce material that may initially seem tangential or unimportant, and control the tempo, pace, and movement of the story. Responding to the narrator with genuine curiosity and requests for more detailed elaboration communicates interest and supports a mutual process of discovery. Narrative-friendly questions ask for concrete and particular examples, question the significance of particular events or how choices were made, and elicit the narrator's understanding of causal relationships.

As we listen mindfully, we shall hear stories of love and commitment, of God, of trouble, of power or loss of power, of the meaning of illness and death. We shall hear stories of family, of transitions, of pets, of work and play, of joy and sadness and of expectations. Many stories will embody spiritual issues – the need to give or receive forgiveness, the need to reconnect with a loved one, the laying of blame for illness and death, the pain of being unloved or being unable to love, the guilt for the many things said or unsaid. And there will be questions. *Does God exist? Where is God now? Why is God punishing me? Why me? Why now? What will happen to my family? What has my life meant?*

The greatest gift that we can give to the dying person is to be there, be fully present, and know that our willingness to listen to their stories goes far toward relieving their suffering. Their stories and questions may take many twists and turns, and many may focus on their present situation, but keep in mind that every person has a past and a future – it is not only the present circumstance that should take center stage. We can encourage stories of the past: *What was important? Where did you find joy and contentment? What shaped your life and person or family?* As for the future: *What are your hopes and preferences? What practical problem is facing you? What do you need? How can I help?*

EXERCISES

A. (40 minutes) *Interviews with Family and Friends*

The assignment from Unit 4.3 was to interview two or three friends or family members about how they view death, and which of Lief's patterns best fit their viewpoints and why. All of the participants should share their findings.

B. (20 minutes) Recalling *The Death of Ivan Ilyich*

For the first few minutes, each person should write responses to the following questions. Then discuss the responses in the large group.

You will remember that in the final days and hours of Ivan Ilyich's dying, he reviewed his life. Why did he do this? What spiritual questions was he asking?

Which of Lief's patterns of death assumptions fits Ivan Ilyich best?

____

____

____

____

____

C. (30 minutes) *Spiritual Questions and Statements*

On the following lines, write at least four spiritual questions or statements that you, as a caregiver, think you might hear from a dying person, how you would respond to them, and how it would feel to respond. Then form groups of three or four and discuss your questions/statements and your responses. Share your thoughts with the large group.

____

____

____

____

____

____

____

____

____

____

____

____

D. (40 minutes) *A Story About Dying*

Your trainer will ask for a volunteer to read the following story by James Sturm (4: 301–2) aloud, slowly and with feeling. As you read along and listen, visualize the room, the sights, sounds, smells, and the individuals. When finished, discuss the story and the questions that follow in the large group.

"I'VE NEVER DONE THIS BEFORE"

James L Sturm, D.Min.
Marietta Memorial Hospital
Marietta, Ohio

"Am I going to die today?" she whispers. The afternoon sunlight streams across the room. The head of her rented hospital bed is situated toward the window, and the soft blue of a late winter's sky gives a tenderness to the setting.

"Maybe," I answer. "Are you worried about dying?"

"No, not worried," she replies. "I'd just like to know."

I say, "I guess only God knows."

Silence fills the room and drifts down the hallway. Not long ago this was a spare room used for storage. Now it's the dying room. A small TV sits atop a table in one corner. Its blank screen reflects the view through the window. A tape player and several cassettes lie on a side stand, with a Bible close by. Sometimes the TV is left on to flicker through long nights with its sound muted, while gospel music wafts gently through the air.

On the wall hangs a blue straw hat with white lace, a picture of a kitten, and a round white clock with black numbers. In another corner sits a small night stand, its top covered with medicine and such. The room is cluttered with things.

I pick up her Bible and begin to read softly, "The Lord is my shepherd ..." She sighs and closes her eyes. I count her respirations. Twenty-four. *Not bad, I think to myself. I don't have to hold her wrist to take her pulse.* Her body shakes with every heartbeat. Eighty. That's okay, too. "I shall dwell ... forever ... " Her days seem without end. Her nights, too, and they are filled with dreams so frightful that she tries to stay awake all the time.

I sit in an old brown recliner that had once been discarded to the basement. With silver duct tape covering the wear and tear on the arms, it works well as a place to rest. She opens her eyes and stares toward the wall. Her statements are often irrelevant and incoherent. This disease seems to course through every fiber of her being, and even appears to touch her soul.

"What are you thinking?" I ask.

"My treasures," she whispers, as she gestures toward the things that hang on the wall. Trinkets. Souvenirs of family vacations. Dust collectors. But each one represents a part of her living. Each one has an accompanying story. She tells me some of the stories. They are her stories and no one else's. I listen.

Listening is what she so desperately needs now. All day and all night the listeners come and go. Some tell her not to talk about dying – but that is where she is. She must talk about her dying – and so I listen to her story, and to her dying.

"Are you afraid?" I ask.

"No." she whispers. "It's just that I've never done this before and I don't quite know how to do it." We laugh together. This is part of living, too. The very last part. Silence again envelops the room as we wait together.

QUESTIONS

1. What were your feelings as you read through the story?
2. What picture did you get of the woman (age, physical being, etc.)?
3. How would you describe the feeling between the two individuals?
4. What feelings and sensations did you get of the room?
5. What do you think of the way the minister responded to the dying woman?
6. How would you respond?
7. The minister asked some questions. Were they open-ended or closed? What was he trying to do with his questions?
8. Did the minister hold an open space for the woman? How?
9. What would you have liked to ask her?
10. Have you heard individuals say "Oh, don't talk about that now ... think about something else"? What does that do to the ill person?
11. What did you think about the ending?

(5 MINUTES) REFLECTION ON THIS UNIT

Journal Note for Unit 4.4

____

____

____

____

____

ASSIGNMENT

Read Unit 4.5 and complete Exercise B. Choose one of the expressive activities described there to demonstrate to the group how it can be used to aid the suffering of a dying person. Bring all of the materials you will need with you to the next session.

ADDITIONAL RESOURCES

1. Barnard D, Towers A, Boston P *et al. Crossing Over: narratives of palliative care*. Oxford: Oxford University Press; 2000.
2. Moller DW. *Dancing with Broken Bones: portraits of death and dying among inner-city poor*. Oxford: Oxford University Press; 2004.

REFERENCES

1. Romanoff BD, Thompson BE. Meaning construction in palliative care: the use of narrative, ritual, and the expressive arts. *Am J Hospice Palliat Care Med*. 2006; **23:** 309–16.
2. Cassel EJ. The nature of suffering and the goals of medicine. *N Engl J Med*. 1982; **306:** 639–45.
3. Levine S. *Healing Into Life and Death*. New York: Anchor Book/Doubleday; 1987.
4. Sturm JL. I've never done this before. *J Pastoral Care*. 1998; **52:** 301–2.

Unit 4.5: Expressive Activities That Aid in Relieving Suffering

KEY ISSUES

Music, writing, art forms, literature, symbols, rituals, altars, meditation, prayer.

(10 minutes) Meditation

(10 minutes) Journal Note Share

> *Dying is not a passive act. Viewed as part of living, dying is an opportunity for the last stages of growth – to complete life well and prepare to meet death with peace of mind.*
>
> Christine Longaker (1: 34)

INTRODUCTION

You have learned that for most people who are dying, particularly those who linger in the dying process, suffering may well be part of the journey. And as much as we would like to take their hand and lead them along the path, we understand that the search for meaning and hope cannot be imposed externally. Again, we emphasize that none of us are saviors. It is up to the dying person to do the necessary work to complete life well and find peace of mind. The most we can do is to provide an open and safe space where the dying can grieve their losses, shed their tears, express their fears and concerns, and mend their own souls. You have learned the basic skills that will help to create that open and safe space, namely attending to body language, practicing mindful presence and mindful listening, and responding with empathy.

Outside of what you bring personally to the relationship there are some other techniques and expressive activities that you can introduce to the dying person, such as music, writing, art, etc., that may help them to open emotional and spiritual space in the following ways:

- alter the perception of physical pain
- promote muscular relaxation
- encourage emotional release
- improve sleep
- lessen the sense of isolation
- encourage spiritual strengthening
- clarify cultural beliefs
- strengthen family bonds
- reinforce identity and self-worth
- explore the need to give and receive forgiveness.

In this Unit we shall explore several different activities and interventions, and we rely on the creative nature of participants to design other techniques that might be helpful. **A word of caution**: any approach to relieving suffering must be co-created with the dying person, who must not feel coerced or uncomfortable in any way. Furthermore, the caregiver must remember that, for some individuals, suffering has spiritual meaning and purpose. This most certainly may be explored, but it must not be judged or devalued.

Music

Greenstreet (2: 153) writes that "Music is primordial within us all, at the very heart of our existence, the reason why man, for millennia, has used music as a means to enhance well-being." Throughout the ages and in all cultures, music, sound, and rhythm have been used in ministering to the sick. From the Renaissance period there are accounts of the influence of music on breathing, blood pressure, muscular activity, and digestion (3). Through our own experience we know that music touches feelings and moods that words and medicines cannot. It can soothe, uplift, and inspire, or it can irritate. It can elicit spiritual memories and feelings, or powerful and conflicting negative emotions. It can generate doubt and anxiety or it can promote healing. Selected by the dying person and used fittingly, music can promote relaxation and soothe anxieties.

Writing

Writing has a very particular power in that it enables us to understand ourselves better – what we think, what we know, what we don't know, and what we feel. Writing can be profoundly therapeutic (4). It can provide a release of hidden feelings about death, it can convey last wishes or requests, and it is a way to affirm life's meaning and purpose. Writing can take any form – a short essay or poem, letters to loved ones, a journal, creation of lifelines and timelines, or writing one's own obituary, funeral plans, or eulogy. All are effective means of connecting with loved ones and gaining understanding and easing tension.

Other Art Forms

Paintings, photographs, sculpture, glass art, wood art, and other art forms can positively affect mood, summon happy memories and soothe fears. Some favorites may be found in the person's home, or the caregiver might offer to locate them outside the home. Encouraging the dying person to create their own art form is particularly effective. This would require art supplies to be available.

Literature

Reading certain favorite literary works or poetry is often soothing for the dying person. Scripture and other sacred texts may also provide solace, particularly if they are favorites chosen by the dying person.

Symbols and Rituals

We all keep symbols around us – gifts from loved ones, pictures, clothing, art pieces, children's first writings, etc. – that represent comforting reminders of love, work, and family. For the dying person, symbols are emotionally charged materials that maintain connections to a life that is ending. We envisioned the many symbols that belonged to the elderly woman in the story in Unit 4.4. Encouraging the dying person to share the meaning of the symbols helps to affirm life's meaning. Likewise, helping the dying person to create a memory book containing symbols of their life, such as pictures, stories, poems, or children's artwork, can be very gratifying and affirming.

"Rituals," as they are described by Romanoff and Thompson (5: 312), "are deliberate, detailed, and repeated patterns of activity that are infused with multiple meaning. They serve to reaffirm social ties, mark changes in identity, generate meaning that fosters a sense of solidarity, and manage crises." Reflecting on the authors' words, we can see that rituals can have great value for the dying person. Personalized and creative rituals can help individuals to complete unfinished business and promote for themselves and their loved ones a sense of peace, reconciliation, and acceptance.

Altars

An altar can be merely a gathering of significant, heartwarming symbols positioned to create a *sacred space* anywhere in the dying person's room or home – on a bedside table, on top of a bureau, on a table in a comfortable corner of the room, or perhaps on a window ledge. An altar focuses consciousness on the spirit, and embodies the notion of communion and love.

Meditation

At this point in this training program, you have become very familiar with the practice and forms of meditation. You have learned that meditations are chosen to meet certain purposes, and that they should be practiced regularly if they are to be beneficial. All forms of meditation help to quiet the mind and foster mindfulness. Most meditative techniques place a focus on the breath, and some include music, rhythm, or movement. Research has shown considerable medical benefit from the regular practice of meditation and meditative forms such as meditative walking, yoga, or Tai Chi. It is especially useful in the control of pain and for improving sleep (6–8).

Prayer

Clearly, prayer is a highly personal experience. We recognize that organized faith traditions have specific prayer rituals, but it must be remembered that they may or may not be practiced by the dying person. It is not appropriate, and is perhaps even unethical, for a caregiver to initiate prayer with the dying person without their consent and without the dying person describing the purpose of the prayer. As for the caregiver who is not of the same faith, they may feel uncomfortable when asked to lead prayer, read a passage, or even to participate in prayer. In these instances, the caregiver should remember that being present during the other's prayer or reading a favorite passage does not indicate belief in that faith. Rather, it is evidence of a supportive and caring relationship. Caregivers can refer to chaplains and clergy for help with this activity.

EXERCISES

A. (30 minutes) *Symbols and Rituals*

For the first 5 minutes, write your responses to the following questions, then form small groups of three or four and share your responses. Briefly share some thoughts in the large group.

Describe the symbols that you keep around you. What meaning do they have for you? What effect do they have on you?

____

____

____

____

____

____

Describe the rituals that you observe in your daily life and the meaning that they have for you.

Describe the rituals that are part of your spiritual life and the meaning that they have for you.

Describe the rituals that help you to maintain your relationships with family members or friends.

B. (100 minutes) *Expressive Activities Demonstrations*

This is the assignment from Unit 4.4. Each participant was instructed to choose an activity described in the Unit to demonstrate to the group, and describe how the technique is helpful. (For example, "This activity is useful in that it tends to relax the muscles and therefore reduces physical pain.") Share your interventions with the large group.

(5 MINUTES) REFLECTIONS ON THIS UNIT

Journal Note for Unit 4.5

____

____

____

____

____

ASSIGNMENT

(To be determined by the trainer.)

ADDITIONAL RESOURCES

1. Aldridge D, ed. *Music Therapy in Palliative Care: new voices*. London: Jessica Kingsley Publishers; 2001.
2. Elias J. *Prayer Cycle*. Sony Music Entertainment, Inc.; 1999.
3. Myss C. *Chakra Meditation Music*. Boulder, CO: Sounds True, Inc.; 2002.
4. Stillwater M, Malken GR, producers. *Graceful Passages: a companion for living and dying*. Novato, CA: Companion Arts; 2000.
5. Schroeder-Sheker T. *Rosa Mystica*. Tucson, AZ: Celestial Harmonics; 1990.
6. Evanson E, Barabas T. *Wind Dancer*. Tuczon, AZ: Sounds of the Planet; 1992.
7. Feldman MG. *Hospice Music*. Andover, MA: Cool Biz Productions; 2000.
8. Voces Novae. *Meditations on Life–Death*. Clear Creek, IN; Voces Novae; 2001.

REFERENCES

1. Longaker C. *Facing Death and Finding Hope: a guide to the emotional and spiritual care of the dying*. London: Century; 1997.
2. Greenstreet W. *Integrating Spirituality in Health and Social Care*. Oxford: Radcliffe Publishing; 2006.
3. Munro S, Mount B. Music therapy in palliative care. *CMA Journal*. 1978; **119:** 1029–34.
4. Bolton G. Writing is a way of saying things I can't say and didn't know I knew. In: *Proceedings of the Seventh Humanism and the Healing Arts Conference*, Institute for Professionalism Institute, Summa Health System, Akron, OH. April 2008.
5. Romanoff BD, Thompson BE. Meaning construction in palliative care: the use of narrative, ritual, and the expressive arts. *Am J Hospice Palliat Care*. 2006; **23:** 309–16.
6. Kabat-Zinn J, Massion AO, Kresteller J *et al.* Effectiveness of meditation-based stress reduction program on the treatment of anxiety disorders. *Am J Psychiatry*. 1992; **149:** 136-43.
7. Kabat-Zinn J, Litworth L, Buaney R *et al.* Four-year follow-up of a meditation-based program for self-regulation of chronic pain and treatment outcomes and compliance. *J Pain*. 1986; **2:** 159–73.
8. Reibel DK, Greeson JM, Gainor GC *et al.* Mindfulness-based stress reduction and health-related quality of life in a heterogeneous patient population. *Gen Hosp Psychiatry*. 2001; **23:** 183–92.

Part 5:
Honoring the Caregiver

Being a caregiver for a dying person, whether it is your full-time professional career, or the role you fulfill in your home for someone you love, or the commitment you have made as a volunteer, is a courageous and commendable undertaking. You may well find that it becomes one of the richest and most meaningful experiences of your life. However, as we noted earlier, it may also be one of the most draining and sobering. **Finding ways to honor and care for yourself is vital in caregiving**.

This chapter provides you with the opportunity to explore ways to keep yourself physically, emotionally, and spiritually healthy. It asks you to conduct a final self-check on your readiness to be an effective caregiver, and to create a set of criteria that will serve as guidelines for you as you make the journey with a dying person.

Unit 5.1: Nurture and Honor Yourself!

KEY ISSUES

Self-care, readiness for caregiving, caregiver oath.

(10 minutes) Meditation

(10 minutes) Journal Note Share

> *Becoming responsible for another's care takes courage as well as energy, firmness as well as tenderness, self-discipline as well as self-sacrifice.*
>
> James E. Miller (1: 5)

> *The truth is that we all fall off of our clarity, our calm, our balance, our openness of heart, time and time again. Self-care is the act of re-aligning ourselves with the stream of life in ways that return us to our gifts of immediate living, especially when we are confused, agitated, out of balance, or closed.*
>
> Mark Nepo (2: 31)

INTRODUCTION

We have arrived at the end of this training program. You have worked hard, gained new knowledge, learned many new skills, and are prepared to embark upon a journey with a dying person. It is a great privilege to be invited to share the last days of someone's life, to hold their hand and ease their spirit. You may still harbor some anxiety about your readiness or your ability, but it is time to put your fears behind you and move forward. Whether you are a professional caregiver, a relative, or a hospice or palliative care volunteer, caring for a dying person can be demanding both emotionally and physically. During this time, caring for oneself becomes paramount.

The following story (3), *Giving Care*, written by Ronna Edelstein, poignantly describes the trials and tribulations of caring for her aging parents, and her underlying need, in Nepo's words, to "realign herself with the stream of life." One or more participants should volunteer to read the following story.

Giving Care

When I was six, my family and I spent a week in Atlantic City. I loved the Boardwalk with its saltwater-taffy aroma and colorful sights, but I feared the pier that jutted out into the Atlantic. One moonless night, my big brother bet me a bag of taffy that I couldn't walk to the pier's end by myself. Never one to back down, I accepted his bet. But the further out I walked, the more frightened I got. It felt like one more step would send me off the pier's edge and into the bottomless black water. My parents rescued me by dashing to the end of the pier and carrying me back to safety.

I spent the next half-century living under two illusions: one, that nothing in my life would ever be as scary as that dark pier; and two, that my parents would always be there to save me. In school, when my Lilliputian classmates mocked my five-foot-eight-inch stature, Ma and Dad talked to me about inner beauty and strength. After the rice strewn along my wedding aisle disintegrated into sharp slivers of divorce, Ma and Dad gave me the financial and emotional support I needed to raise my son and daughter.

When after thirty-five years I returned to my hometown of Pittsburgh, I hosted Sunday-night dinners for my parents and ran errands for them. Yet they still saw me as their little girl; whether stocking my refrigerator or slipping mad money into my wallet, they made sure that I was okay. I found a balance between spending time with them and going out to dinners, movies and plays with my new circle of friends. Life was good.

Then, four years ago, like Alice, I tumbled into a topsy-turvy world. My eyes finally saw what my heart had refused to acknowledge: Ma was losing her mental edge. No longer was she the formidable woman who'd kept a spotless house and worked at a children's furniture store.

And Dad, on our long walks, was leaning more and more on his cane and my arm for support.

My parents, once my constant caregivers, now needed me to be theirs. As a result, I've spent the past four years feeling as if I'm once again tottering towards the pier's end – this time with no rescue in sight. To make room for Ma and her dementia and Dad and his aging, I willingly relinquished the starring role in my own life, feeling that as they had so willingly given to me, I should give to them.

Being an educator, I initially tried to embrace caregiving as a learning experience. Trying to feed Ma pieces of chocolate-chip cookies, I immediately halted when she whispered "I can feed myself," reminding me that, even with dementia, she was still my mother, not a child.

I quickly realized that caregiving can be a harsh teacher. I had to make difficult decisions, placing Ma in an assisted-living facility, and giving up my apartment to move in with Dad.

And day-to-day caregiving, I discovered, is a powerful mix of deep satisfaction and profound irony. As Ma passively let me change her dirty diapers and urine-soaked bed sheets, I found myself resenting the distasteful tasks and mourning the feisty, capable woman I'd so admired. And when she mistook me for her sister, or a total stranger, I couldn't rationalize away my hurt, Other times, we would enjoy a moment of grace when she held my face in her hands and called me by name.

When Ma died in my arms in March 2007, a part of me rejoiced that she was finally at peace. Another part wondered if I myself could ever find peace and whether I'd done my very best for her.

Life with Dad – physically weakened but mentally sound at ninety-three – offers its own highs and lows. Often my one and only wish is that our life together would never change. I love taking him to the mall for lunch or to the park for an afternoon of people-watching. Every night I massage his arthritic legs; every Saturday we travel back in time together, watching *The Lawrence Welk Show.*

Although Dad encourages me to spend time with friends, he gets despondent and frightened when I do make plans. So I've had to ask friends' understanding for my dwindling availability, and my once-full calendar is now rows of blank spaces.

I loathe my friends' emails describing "must-see" movies or plays that I probably won't. And I resent my brother when it feels like he's able to visit Paris and London but somehow can't manage the twenty-minute drive to see Dad.

At night I toss and turn, as if trying to claw my way out of this rabbit hole that has swallowed my life. I sometimes vent my pent-up feelings with a therapist friend or use my iPod music or treadmill walks to calm down. But, like a child worried that stepping on a crack will break a parent's back, I try to avoid complaining for fear that some avenging angel will take Dad from me.

And time, like Alice's White Rabbit, keeps racing ahead.

Sometimes I fantasize awakening one morning to discover, like Alice, that my experiences have been a dream, and that Ma and Dad are their old selves again. But deep down I know that, instead, someday I'll find myself truly alone at the end of the pier.

When that happens, I hope that the lessons I've worked hard on as a caregiver – patience and perseverance, acceptance of unplanned moments, tolerance of change, kindness towards myself and others – will stick with me and help to steady and support me as I step forward into my new life.

If you, like Ms. Edelstein, are caring for a dying person at home, in addition to your usual daily responsibilities – your work and your family – you may also be providing nursing care as well as daily nourishment and emotional comfort and support. You have a heavy and tiring load. For the professional caregiver, there are other patients and staff to care for and the added responsibilities for paperwork, meetings, and administrative duties. In both of these circumstances, caregiving is draining and often confusing and worrisome. Without adequate self-care, burnout is inevitable. Even for lay volunteers, although the responsibilities may be fairly limited and far less demanding of time, the psycho-emotional impact can be significant. Caring for yourself is not a selfish act. It's a matter of replenishing your energy, maintaining your health, and renewing your spirit so that you can continue your efforts. Miller's advice (1: 13) is to become aware of and to satisfy your own personal needs:

- Find ways to get the rest you cannot do without, however strong you are, and however loving you feel.
- Maintain your energy by eating healthily and drinking wisely. Build your stamina by exercising regularly.
- Make sure you set aside time each day just for yourself.
- Open yourself to healing influences all around you – through prayer and meditation, nature, art, music, and literature.
- Allow yourself opportunities for fun.
- Indulge yourself from time to time.
- Engage in those practices that expand your mind and touch your soul.
- Remember that *only* by caring for yourself can you adequately care for another.

EXERCISES

A. (30 minutes) *Readiness to be a Caregiver*

For the first 5 minutes, write your responses to the questions on the lines below. Share your responses with a partner and then with the large group.

What knowledge, skills, attitudes, and behaviors do you believe you possess that will enable you to be an effective caregiver?

____

____

____

____

____

Describe and explain how you feel regarding your readiness to attend a dying person.

____

____

____

Describe how you think you will feel on your first visit to a dying person.

B. (30 minutes) *Caring for Myself*

On the lines below, write down the ways in which you will care for yourself while you are caring for another. Share these with the large group.

C. (60 minutes) *Caregiver's Oath*

You are ready to begin the journey. Form small groups of three or four and write the statements that you believe should be included in a Caregiver's Oath. This will provide you with a summary of the guidelines for caregiving. With a marker pen write your statements on chart paper and mount this on a nearby wall for everyone to see. Compare the statements from all of the groups. Construct one Oath for the large group. You will repeat this Oath during your commencement exercises.

Caregivers' Oath

____

____

____

____

____

____

____

(5 MINUTES) REFLECTION ON UNIT 5.1

Journal Note for Unit 5.1

____

____

____

____

REFERENCES

1. Miller JE. *The Caregiver's Book: caring for another, caring for yourself.* Minneapolis, MN: Augsburg Fortress; 1996.
2. Nepo M. Falling off and beginning again. In: *Proceedings of the Eighth Humanism and the Healing Arts Conference*, Institute for Professionalism Inquiry, Summa Health System, Akron, OH, October 2008: 30–36.
3. Edelstein CL. Pulse. www.pulsemagazine.org (accessed 2 July 2009).

For Product Safety Concerns and Information please contact our EU
representative GPSR@taylorandfrancis.com
Taylor & Francis Verlag GmbH, Kaufingerstraße 24, 80331 München, Germany

www.ingramcontent.com/pod-product-compliance
Ingram Content Group UK Ltd.
Pitfield, Milton Keynes, MK11 3LW, UK
UKHW050832080625
459435UK00015B/592

* 9 7 8 1 8 4 6 1 9 3 8 4 2 *